Our Children Are...

What Our Children Eat

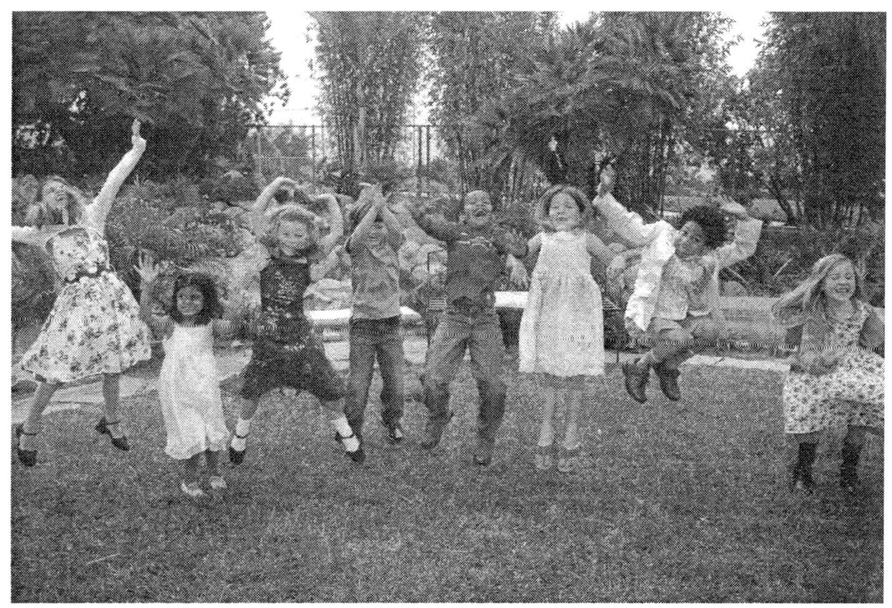

Nutritional Solutions for Improving Behavior, Health and School Performance

By Dr. Laura Thompson

The information in this book is intended to be helpful and educational. It is not meant to be diagnostic or prescriptive, or to replace the advice of a qualified health care professional. Use your own good judgment and consult with your chosen medical or health care practitioner when planning your family health program.

Cover photograph of the children from Wisdom for Life School, *Encinitas, California* **by Monique Feil,** www.moniquefeil.com

Cover art by Wm. Michael Mott, www.mottimorphic.com

The Library of Congress has catalogued this edition as follows:
Thompson PhD, Laura N.
Library of Congress Control Number 2008922369
ISBN: 1-93-1359032

 Published by America's House of Health, Encinitas, CA 92024, info@ourchildrenshealth.com.

This book is dedicated to my husband, Jon Rappoport, and my parents, Maenelle and Dick Thompson.

Many thanks to Sue Toftee, Theresa Caprio, Barbara Keeler, Dr. John Taylor, Lawrence Greb, Linda Ochwat, Cathie Flickner, Lesley DeLuz and Lisa Boyd for their expertise and support.

About Dr. Laura Thompson

Dr. Laura Thompson is the CEO and founder of the Southern California Institute of Clinical Nutrition located in Carlsbad, California and the IN Solutions Apothecary. Dr. Thompson received her Ph.D. in Nutrition and Human Behavior from Ryokan College in Los Angeles, California, studied naturopathy and iridology with Dr. Bernard Jensen, and culinary arts at the Paris American Academy in Paris, France. She is board certified in Naturopathic Endocrinology by the American Naturopathic Certification and Accreditation Board and has helped thousands of men & women through natural health and hormone programs.

Dr. Thompson has an international phone consulting practice, with clients in 7 countries and all 50 of the United States. Her specialties are hormonal, brain and digestive health and she is an avid proponent of natural medicine and super food nutrition as a means of family wellness, weight management and longevity. Dr. Thompson designs lab-based nutritional and naturopathic programs to help people overcome a wide variety of health problems and achieve optimum well-being and vitality.

Her books and newsletters inspire, educate and motivate families, including families of children with ADD, ADHD and autism to positively transform behavior, health, athletic and academic performance. She is a popular lecturer at autism and ADHD conferences in North America, on topics such as Natural Solutions for ADHD and Natural Hormone Programs for Men, Women and Teens.

In addition, she is an instructor at the Natural Healing Institute of Naturopathy in Encinitas, California, teaching nutrition and natural hormone classes to future health practitioners. Dr. Thompson is a member of the nutritional and medical advisory boards for Simplexity Health International, Nutrition and Kids (NAKA), America's House of Health, the Synergy Foundation and the Truth Seeker Company. She is also the founder of the IN Solutions Apothecary in Carlsbad, California.

Dr. Thompson has been a guest on radio and TV shows nationwide, and is the author of:

- Book: *Smart Food, Smart Families* - Recipes and techniques for growing families
- CD: A New Life: Return to Balance - Natural hormone programs for men and women
- CD: The Great Defender - Nutritional solutions for immune system strength
- E-mail newsletter - Nutrition World Online (scicn.com)

Dr. Thompson is also a contributing writer for various trade magazines and other publications such as the Natural Food Merchandiser, Whole Life Times, and several independent online newsletters. She is currently working on informational CD's and several books, soon to be published. She is married to Jon Rappoport, author, investigative reporter and artist; they live in Encinitas, California. Dr. Thompson consults with people worldwide through phone consultations or individual in-office visits.

Dr. Laura Thompson can be reached for private nutritional consultations:

Southern California Institute of Clinical Nutrition
(800) 608-5602
www.scicn.com
www.ourchildrenshealth.com
www.insolutions.info

Introduction

I wrote this book to empower the people who help the children. My purpose is to help achieve peace at home and peace in the classroom.

From infancy through teen years, health problems are rampant. 17% of children and adolescents between ages 2 and 19 years are overweight. Childhood obesity and diabetes are on the rise, and children are saddled with with acid reflux, skin and respiratory disorders, high cholesterol, as well as mild and severe depression. Kids are more aggressive and violent now than ever. They don't feel good.

The CDC, Centers for Disease Control, reports that 7.8% of the children in the U.S. are diagnosed with Attention Deficit Disorder. 56% of them are being treated with medication. ADD/ADHD is the #1 psychiatric disorder among children. Do you believe they – our children, our students -- are all sick and have mental diseases? Or are many of them falsely diagnosed and under-nourished?

We have a health industry that loves to diagnose, a public who is eager for the diagnosis and a multi-billion dollar industry that loves to sell drugs.

The health problems children ARE having are being over-drugged, and the problems they DON'T have are being diagnosed as diseases or disorders.

Then there are the food corporations. Trends come and go at the speed of light. Kids are subject to commercialization far beyond our comprehension. The "market" has turned them into consumers and "users" – of toys, of devices, of food and drink.

Most of the children in North America today are eating the same commercial foods – low in nutrients and high in calories: sodas, juice drinks, macaroni and cheese, pizza, sugary cereals, French fries, chicken nuggets, candy and ice cream. Eating these empty foods day in and day out causes a whole range of health problems.

Yes, we have wonderful experts and diagnostic tools with which to assess imbalances, but could it be that something so simple -- nutritional gaps, missing nutrients -- are a major factor in what's happening to our kids? You will find many scientific studies in this book that validate this concept. You will also read about numerous solutions.

These solutions are drug-free and at our fingertips. But you have to reach out of the box, because that's where the answers are. Answers to: over-medicating; over-diagnosing; missing nutrients; addictive eating. Answers to a whole range of children's health problems that have come looming up over the horizon.

Parents, grandparents, teachers, and other caregivers have found answers for their children's health and they are living them. It is so inspiring to watch them transform children's lives – on their own --- by their own decision, by their own doing --- with just some information --- like the information that follows.

Thank you for reading.

Dr. Laura Thompson

Table of Contents

PART ONE - THE FOUNDATION:

How We're Made, What We Need to Grow

Chapter One

OUR CHILDREN'S HEALTH

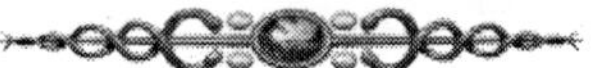

This book is about problems and solutions for the many aspects of children's health. Moreover, it reveals the real causes of the problems – nothing white-washed. In order to understand the solutions, we first have to know what the problems are. This chapter is designed to do just that – expose the truth, the facts, the statistics.

Know though, that the solutions are close behind. They are many and varied – because each child is unique. There is no one magic bullet. Children heal; get balanced physically, mentally and emotionally with good food, good air, good water and good sense.

It is likely that if you are reading this book, the studies, and the scientific evidence in this chapter will be of interest to you. Studies like these are usually listed in the back of a book – too small to read. They are, however, far too important to treat that way, so I have given them a prominent place.

Pediatric Diseases Are Epidemic

There has been a tremendous rise in many physical as well as mental and emotional health conditions in children today. Many of these diseases are chronic, requiring ongoing care. Chronic can also imply activity-limiting. Children's lives are restricted due to symptoms of their conditions:

- breathing problems
- fatigue
- social maladaptation
- anxiety
- pain

Obesity takes center stage in studies about chronic diseases in children today. ADHD and asthma/allergies are not far behind:

Increase in Overweight Girls and Boys
Ogden, CL, PhD; et al "Prevalence of Overweight and Obesity in the United States, 1999-2004", *JAMA*, 2006; 295:1549-1555.

From 1990-2004: Overweight in girls increased from 13.8% to 16.0%
Overweight in boys increased from 14.0% to 18.2%.

ADHD, Asthma, Obesity in Children, On the Rise
Perrin, JM. MD; Bloom, SR, MS; Gortmaker, SL, PhD, "The Increase of Childhood Chronic Conditions in the U.S.", *Journal of American Medical Association*, 2007; 297:2755-2759

-Obesity, asthma & ADHD are driving the growth of chronic illnesses.
-Chronic activity-limiting conditions rose 1.8% to 7% from 1960-2004.
-Childhood obesity, at 18%, has quadrupled in the last 30 years.
-Almost 60% of 5- to 10-year-old obese children have one associated cardiovascular disease risk factor. More than 20% have 2 or more risk factors.
-An estimated 9% of children have asthma, double what it was in the 1980s.

Rising ADHD Diagnosis and Use of Meds
Report on the "Prevalence of Diagnosed and Medicated ADHD: US, 2003", CDC, Sept 20, 2005

The CDC reports that ADHD diagnosis occurs in 7.8% of school-aged children. 2.5 million Youth, ages 4-17, were receiving medication treatment for ADHD.

This is the first generation of children who have been brought up with so many nutrient deficiencies, resulting from a variety of problems ----- with the soil, with nutrient-depleted food, and with heavily chemical-laden foods. We are now seeing only the beginning of the consequences of these hazards. There are more degenerative and neurological illnesses in children now, than ever -- encephalopathies, epilepsy, convulsions, autism, mental retardation and central nervous system disorders. Learning disabilities are rampant.

And the illnesses are developing at very young ages. The increase of these diseases in children is staggering. Emotional, behavioral and developmental problems have skyrocketed in the last years, as seen in the following study:

2003 National Survey of Children's Health in America
"Emotional, developmental et al, Banchard LT Gurka MJ, Blackman JA, *Journal of Pediatrics*, 2006 June; 117(6) el202-12)

The most commonly diagnosed emotional, developmental and behavioral problems among children 6-17 years of age:
-- Learning disabilities – 11.5%
-- ADHD – 8.8%
-- Behavioral problems – 6.3%
-- Speech problems – 5.8%
-- Developmental delays – 3.2%

Is there common ground here? Yes, most of the children are exposed to an incredible toxic load – from vaccinations, antibiotics and chemicals in their food. And many health conditions and diseases are perpetuated by eating toxic food. There is little chance of disease reversal or swift recovery without the building blocks from good food.

So, it isn't bad parenting or bad teaching --- it's bad food! Most kids today are eating the same foods: sugary cereals, school lunches, pizza, burgers and fries, sodas, red, green, and blue drinks, and macaroni and cheese out of a box. They can't sustain their lives this way --- not vibrant, healthy lives, at least, not for long.

Parents as Teachers

Parents always were and always will be a child's most important teachers. So much important information about nutrition and eating can come from the home. Healthy eating should be a family affair. Kids eat what they are taught to eat. Teach them to eat healthy food and show them by example. Help them see the benefits of eating healthy food – primarily, feeling good and preventing illness. Knowledge is power. What we teach our children now, they will know forever.

Kids and Adults Positively Respond to Learning about Fruits and Veggies

Haire-Joshu D, Elliott MB, et al. High 5 for Kids: "The impact of a home visiting program on fruit and vegetable intake of parents and preschool children." *Amer Journ Prev Med*, July 2008, 47(1):77-82.

-- This study revolved around the idea that Parents Are Teachers.
-- The program focusing on eating veggies and fruits was very successful.
-- Parents increased fruit and veggie consumption, predicting an increase for their child.
-- For every full serving of fruits and veggies for the parent, there was an increase of ½ serving for the child. Parents also reported better knowledge of foods in their home.

Parents as Role Models for Nutrition

Haire-Joshu D, Elliott MB, et al. High 5 for Kids: "The impact of a home visiting program on fruit and vegetable intake of parents and preschool children." *Amer Journ Prev Med*, July 2008, 47(1):77-82.

The impulse to imitate in childhood is very strong. Parents are the role models for their kids and are more successful teaching their kids to eat right when their plate is full of healthy selections. If you're asking your child to eat vegetables and fish while you graze on potato chips and soda, your actions will override your good intentions.

Obese Parents, Obese Kids
"Predicting Obesity in Young Adulthood from Childhood and Parental Obesity", Whitaker, RC, MD, Wright, JA, MD, Pepe, MS, PhD, et al, *New Eng Journal of Medicine*, Volume 337:869-873, Sept 25, 1997, No. 13

Conclusions: If the parents are obese, the risk of the child becoming obese as an adult more than doubles, whether the child is obese or not. Childhood obesity is a predictor of adult obesity, regardless of whether the parents are obese.

Children Eat More Fruits and Vegetables if they're Homegrown
Nanney, M. "Children Eat More Fruits And Vegetables If They Are Homegrown." *Journal of the American Dietetic Association*, April 2007; vol 107: pp 577-584.

Over 1,600 parents of preschool-aged children reported: those who ate homegrown fruits and vegetables were more than twice as likely to eat five servings a day, than those who rarely or never ate homegrown produce. Garden-fed children were more likely to see their parents eating fruits and vegetables.

The more often parents eat out, the less they eat fruits and veggies.

Food is Our Glue

Food tastes good. After eating, we have a sense of fulfillment. Meals also provide communal fulfillments. In fact, food is our glue. When we eat together, we're on the same page – we have a level playing ground. Having a meal in common sets the stage for the phrase – "the whole is greater than the sum of its parts." A good meal together can provide good food, good nutrients, good conversation, shared responsibilities (have the kids help with preparation), mutual decisions, laughter and unity.

Eat outside the box – take a picnic dinner to the park, have barbecue night, ethnic food night, such as Greek night with a variety of healthy dips, or fondue night. Avoid distractions such as TV so as to engage in conversation. Use this valuable time to check in with your children. Involve them in the conversation. Listen to them.

Mealtime is also a good opportunity to talk about healthy eating and potential consequences of poor eating habits. Children can relate to: you can grow taller, be stronger, run faster, think better, feel happy, have clear skin and look better.

In actuality though, we eat to live. Plain and simple. Our food must be digested and absorbed into the bloodstream in order to feed our cells. That means the food becomes the cells. The nutrients we absorb – proteins, carbohydrates, fats, vitamins and minerals are what build our bodies. Can you see it that way? If your child has multi-colored, sugary cereal in the morning, then that is what will go into his or her blood stream and attempt to feed the cells. Or if he or she has oatmeal with honey, that is what will go into the bloodstream and feed the cells. Which would you choose?

No matter what is ingested, it circulates throughout the body's heart, liver, brain, and the rest of the organs and glands. This is a big deal. Your food becomes your body, your brain and all your organs.

By getting the necessary proteins, carbohydrates, fats, vitamins, minerals and enzymes into the bloodstream, we have the building blocks for the ongoing turnover of our cells, for growth and repair, energy, metabolism, immune function, brain function, and --- for life!

It is amazing that in this time of high availability of food in North America, our children are malnourished – and not due to lack of quantity, but lack of quality. In the long term this can lead to serious illness; in the short term --- well, we are seeing that now – overweight, unhappy, aggressive, fidgety, anxious, unwell children.

Let's look at some studies so we can isolate where science says some of the problems are, and then let's talk about solutions.

Children Fail to Meet the RDA for Food Groups

"Food intakes of U.S. children & adolescents compared with recommendations", *Pediatrics* 1997 September; 100(3):323-9

A USDA dietary survey of 3,300 U.S. children and adolescents revealed that less than 1% met the RDA for all five food groups.
16% did not meet any of the requirements.

Children's Fat Intake Leads to Obesity and Heart Disease

Nicklas, T.A., Dietary Studies of Children: "The Bogalusa Heart Study Experience", *Journal of American Dietetic Association,* 95:1127-33, 1995

75% of children consume more total fat and saturated fats than the recommended amount. This frightening fact can lead to increased obesity and cardiovascular disease among children and teens.

Children Have Low Fiber Intake

Hempl, J, Betts, N, Benes, B, "The 'Age + 5' Rule: Comparisons of Dietary Fiber Intake among 4-10 Year Olds", *Journal of American Dietetics Association* 1998 December

603 children aged 4-6 years and 782 children aged 7-10 years were told to consume a fiber amount equal to their age plus an additional 5 grams. This is the Age + 5 Rule. About 40% of them consumed adequate fiber.

So 60% of the children did not meet the fiber requirements.
Those who met this rule ate significantly more, high-and low-fiber breads and cereals, fruits, vegetables, legumes, nuts and seeds. Eating fiber-rich foods put these children at a lower risk for future chronic disease.

Declining Fruit and Vegetable Consumption with Kids and Teens

Larson NI, et al. "Trends in adolescent fruit and vegetable consumption", 1999-2004: Project EAT. *American Journal of Preventative Medicine* 32(2), 2007.

From middle school or junior high to high school, teens <u>decreased</u> their intake of fruits and vegetables by almost one serving per day. Girls went from 4 to 3 servings per day. Boy went from 2 ½ to 2 servings per day. From high school to early adulthood, their consumption reduced by almost the same amount. Using processed and fast foods was a major cause of this trend.

More frequent family meals help adolescents eat more healthfully.

The ABC's of Our Children's Bodies

We build, grow and repair our bodies with the food that we eat. Your children's food should be superb, high quality and nutritious. Sometimes we get confused about what that means. Every day we hear that this or that food is all the rage. But, besides new findings and studies, the facts stand for themselves.

Food Falls into 2 Categories

1. Macro nutrition
2. Micro nutrition

Macro nutrition includes: the carbohydrates, proteins and fats and they consist of micronutrients: sugars (starches), amino acids and fatty acids. Micro nutrition also includes vitamins, minerals and enzymes. Seems pretty easy, doesn't it?

It is. However, the quality of foods our children eat makes the difference between health and disease, good brain function and poor brain function, and even between good behavior and poor behavior. It is so important to find the foods that are complete with, and not depleted of, all the macro and micronutrients.

The Macronutrients: Carbohydrates, Proteins and Fats

The carbohydrates are made up of various types of sugars and starches. Common carbohydrate foods are grains, breads, pastas and cereals. Most of them are processed and refined. The better-quality ones are made from whole, unrefined sources. Fruits and vegetables also have carbohydrate content. Our bodies use carbohydrates for energy production.

Proteins are made up of amino acids. Common animal protein foods are dairy products, meats, poultry, eggs and seafood. Proteins from the vegetable kingdom are legumes or beans, soy products, such as tofu and miso, and nuts and seeds. Protein foods help stabilize blood sugar, provide raw materials for the neurotransmitters in the brain, and are necessary for growth and repair of tissues in the body.

Many animal proteins are full of chemicals, such as antibiotics to ward off bacteria in the animals' food and living situations, and added hormones to encourage faster growth and milk production. In fact, most of the toxic chemical residues are found in animal products: meat, poultry, seafood, dairy and eggs. These protein foods can and should be purchased organic, without the drugs and chemicals. The cost is more; the pay-off is even higher.

Fats consist of fatty acids. Common fat foods are oils, butter, whole dairy products, desserts, fast foods, fried foods, avocados, nuts and seeds. The good fats are organic seed and nut oils such as flax, hemp, coconut, walnut, grape seed, apricot kernel, olive and sesame. Other good fats include: avocado and fish oils such as krill oil, salmon oil and cod liver oil.

The Micronutrients: Vitamins, Minerals and Enzymes

The standard definition of micronutrients is: "substances required in the diet only in milligram (mg) or microgram (mcg) amounts, but essential for health and sustaining life." This would include vitamins and minerals. We are, however, including here other micronutrients, as they are the building blocks of macronutrients and are necessary for proper immune function, metabolism, enhanced brain function, digestion and strengthening body tissues.

The micronutrients are:

- **Vitamins** – vital organic nutrients required by plants and animals for life

- **Minerals** – vital nutrients, crystalline in structure and formed by geological processes, necessary for structure and function of plants and animals
- **Enzymes** – protein substances in food that accelerate biochemical activities
- **Fatty acids** – derived from lipids or fats
- **Amino acids** – derived from proteins
- **Glyconutrients** – components of carbohydrates or sugars
- **Phytochemicals** – antioxidants and other substances derived from plants, such as carotenoids or carotenes from green and orange vegetables

These micronutrients are necessary for optimal growth and repair for children. Proper intake of these micronutrients is especially important for children because their primary growth occurs before the age of ten.

Children have different nutritional needs than adults at this time, as rapid growth creates the demand for a daily supply of essential nutrients. The combination of healthy food intake, specific super foods and nutritional supplements help provide the nutrients that children require to develop nerve and brain tissue, muscles, bones, blood and teeth.

Some examples are:

Vitamins A and Beta Carotene

- Support essential growth and development of tissues and bones
- Important for the eyes and all mucous membranes
- Build immunity

B-complex Vitamins

- Balance physical and mental stress
- Maintain a healthy nervous system and brain
- Essential for carbohydrate, protein and fat metabolism

Vitamin C

- Boosts immune function, as a powerful anti-viral
- Provides powerful antioxidant activity, neutralizing free radicals
- Essential for collagen formation

Vitamin D

- Supports absorption of calcium, vital to good teeth & bone development
- Supports the immune system and anti-bacterial, anti-viral activity

Vitamin E

- Supports cellular structures
- Builds hormones
- Heals skin and mucous membranes

Calcium

- Helps manufacture teeth and develop bone
- Balances the nervous system

Magnesium

- Important for calm energy, sleep and muscle health
- Necessary for proper calcium metabolism

Iron

- Support blood cell formation
- Help manufacture neurotransmitters

Zinc

- Heals tissues
- Helps build the enzyme systems
- Important for hormone and neurotransmitter development

Iodine

- Supports thyroid function which impacts metabolism rate and growth

Micronutrients Important for Balanced Brain Chemistry

We are rarely taught about the importance of micronutrients, or vitamins and minerals for proper brain function. In fact, we are told that when we have a brain chemical imbalance, that's just the way it is. *"Can't do anything about it."* But this is totally wrong.

The brain is made of 60% fatty acids. It also functions more efficiently with vitamins and minerals. The brain chemicals are made from amino acids in the presence of vitamins and minerals. These nutrients feed the brain. We **can** change the brain chemistry with specific nutrients and the knowledge about how to use them.

The biological processes of the body such as metabolism and digestion only work in the presence of vitamins and minerals. For instance, magnesium is involved in about 30 amino acid processes, and zinc is involved in over 90 metabolic processes. These functions can only occur with vitamins and minerals. Here's an example:

- The brain chemicals, dopamine and norepinephrine, often deficient in children with attention deficits, require amino acids, vitamin B6 and iron in their pathway in order to be manufactured.
- They also require vitamin C and folic acid.
- If the body does not take in these nutrients, dopamine and norepinephrine will be deficient, and the child's behavior and thinking will be affected.

Micronutrient Deficiencies

It is frightening to think that balanced brain chemistry won't be achieved because certain nutrients are not available. Hear these words – "What we eat affects our brains." I know we're not taught this, but our deficient food is a major culprit here. Because of over-processing, refining and high heat cooking, we have become micronutrient-deficient, low in vitamins, minerals and enzymes.

The vitamins and minerals are also depleted due to over-farmed soil, use of chemical fertilizers, pesticides, and herbicides. In fact, USDA tables of selected foods reveal that we have marked nutrient depletion in our fruits and vegetables today, compared to 20 years ago. They even taste different; they taste empty. Let's remember -- it's the vitamins and minerals that offer the taste – bitter, sweet, sour, salty.

U.S. Senate Document #264 (submitted all the way back in 1936) explains this situation very blatantly:

Deficient Soil, Deficient Bodies

"Proper Food Mineral Balances", *U.S. Senate Doc #264*, 74th Congress 2nd Session, June 1936

"Many states show a marked reduction in the productive capacity of the soil...in many districts amounting to a ***25 to 50 percent reduction in the last 50 years...*** *Some areas show a tenfold variation in calcium. Some show a sixty-fold variation in phosphorous... Authorities...see soil depletion, barren livestock, increased human death rate due to heart disease, deformities, arthritis, increased dental caries, all due to lack of essential minerals in plant foods."*

This problem has gotten progressively worse. Most of our commercial plants are grown in soil with chemical fertilizers that only replace the main 3 out of the 70 minerals. How do we get the other 67? Plants do not manufacture their minerals. They must receive them from the soil. If the soil doesn't have it, it can't pass it along to the plant, and the plant can't pass it along to us.

Most food that can sit on a shelf in a box, can or bag, and not deteriorate, is not worth eating. It is enzyme depleted. It has no life quality if it doesn't mold or "die". It is in effect, already dead. **How can we possibly expect to create vibrant, healthy, alive and exuberant children with dead food?** Remember, their bodies are made from food, air and water. Let's give them good food, good air and good water.

Studies of Specific Nutrient Deficiencies

You'll be amazed about what the following studies reveal: lowered test scores and increased hyperactivity with vitamin and mineral deficiencies. If your doctor or psychologist says there's no scientific proof that nutrition helps in these areas, show them these studies.

Cerebral Function in Iron Deficiency: A Review
Child Care Health Dev, May-June, 1985; 11(3): 105-12

"Children with iron deficiency and anemia show minor defects of cerebral function such as poor attentiveness, poor coordination, and slightly impaired scores on developmental assessments. The patients improved rapidly after treatment with iron."

Magnesium May Decrease Hyperactivity
The Effects of Magnesium Physiological Supplementation on Hyperactivity in Children with ADHD. Positive Response to Magnesium Oral Loading Test. *Magnes Res*, June, 1997; 10(2):149-56

Magnesium deficiency may lead to hyperactivity in children.
Blood and hair magnesium levels were measured with 50 hyperactive children, ages 7-12. Hyperactivity was assessed with both Connor's and Wender's Scales. Results show that children treated with 200 mg. of magnesium for 6 months had a decrease in hyperactivity.

Deficiency of Trace Minerals in Hyperactive Kids
Psychiatr Pol, 1994 May-June; 28(3): 345-53

"The magnesium, zinc, copper, iron and calcium level of plasma, red blood cells, urine, and hair in 50 children aged from 4-13 years with hyperactivity were examined. The average concentration of all trace elements was lower than compared with the control group ---- healthy children. Results show that it is necessary to supplement trace elements in children with hyperactivity."

Is Zinc Deficiency a Public Health Problem?
Nutrition 1995 Jan-Feb; 11 (1 Suppl): 87-92

Women and children are at risk of zinc deficiency, as revealed by comparison of dietary intakes of zinc with requirements. Also, low plasma levels of zinc were associated with abnormal pregnancy outcomes." Controlled trials showed that increasing zinc intake improved pregnancy outcomes. Low zinc was also associated with low iron. "Thus, the hypothesis that zinc deficiency is a public health problem appears to be true."

Relationships Between Serum Fatty Acids and Zinc and ADHD
Bekarolu M, et al. J *Child Psychol* Psychiatry 1996; 37(2):225-7

Forty-eight ADHD and 45 normal children were studied and the ADHD group had significantly lower zinc and fatty acid blood levels.

Vitamin B6 Compared to Ritalin for ADHD
Coleman, M. et al "A Preliminary Study of the Effect of Pyridoxine Administration in a Subgroup of Hyperkinetic Children: A Double-Blind Crossover Comparison with Methylphenidate (Ritalin)" (1979), *Biological Psychiatry*, 14, 741-751.

In a group of subjects with hyperactivity, behavioral improvement with pyridoxine (Vitamin B6) exceeded that with methylphenidate in magnitude, as well as continuation of improvement after cessation of the treatment. There were inconsistent results with the methylphenidate. With B6, blood serotonin levels increased and remained increased after cessation of the treatment, as well as the behavioral improvement.

Essential Fatty Acid (EFA) Metabolism in Boys with ADHD
Stevens L, et al, *Amer. Journal of Clinical Nutrition*, Vol. 62: 761-8, 1995

ADHD boys (assessed by the Connor's Rating Scale) vs. controls showed more thirst, dry hair, ear infections, antibiotic use, asthma, stomach aches. Those with low EFAs (essential fatty acids) showed more allergic rhinitis, temper tantrums, problems at bedtime, thirst and fluid intake. ADHD boys were lower in EFAs, as well as DHA than the non-ADHD control boys.

Essential Fatty Acids Improve Infant IQ
Podell, R, M.D., *Nutrition Science News*, February 1999, vol. 4, No. 2.

Animal experiments show one cause of low intelligence is pre-natal deficiency of essential fatty acids, particularly docosahexaenoic acid (DHA), found in fatty fish and algae supplements. Postnatal studies are also beginning to confirm the connection between DHA and intelligence.

These observations suggest a causative role for essential fatty acid deficiencies in childhood neurological problems. Algae supplements are probably a better source of DHA than EPA for pregnant women.

Relationship of Food & Behavior: Reports & Studies

Below is evidence about the power food has in balancing behavior in children and teens. Teachers, schools and communities have chosen creative solutions:

School Rises Up After Junk-Food Ban
Susie Steiner, *London Times*, May 20, 1999

At Wolsey Junior School in South London, grades and performance improved dramatically after switching from chocolate bars, chips, fizzy drinks and other chemical-laden foods to apples, other fruit and granola bars.

After unhealthy snacks, immediate changes were seen in the concentration and behavior of the students. After the school experienced such success, other teachers, parents and a fruit wholesaler joined together to provide a healthy eating approach.

Diet Change May Avert Need for Ritalin
Jane E. Brody, New York Times, New York, November 2, 1999.

A new report reviews 23 of the best studies conducted since the mid-1970's and public statements from the Food and Drug Administration, the American Academy of Pediatrics, the International Food Information Council and the American Council on Science and Health, among others.

It concludes that the evidence strongly indicates that for some children, behavioral disorders are caused or aggravated by certain food additives, artificial food colors, the foods themselves or a combination.

Applied Nutrition and Behavior
Schoenthaler, SJ, Moody, J, Pankow, L, *Journal of Applied Nutrition*, Nov. 1, 1991, vol. 43.

Review of studies at California State University; implementation of "nutrient dense diets" in 813 state juvenile facilities "resulted in significantly improved conduct, intelligence and/or academic performance..."

Sugar and Hyperactivity
Sucrose: May Cause a Ten Times Increase in Adrenaline Levels in Children Jones, T, Borg W. et al, *Journal of Pediatrics*, Vol 1, 126 (2) Feb 1995, pp. 171 -177.

Sucrose may cause a ten times increase in the stress hormone, adrenaline levels in children resulting in difficulty concentrating, irritability and anxiety.

Diet and Delinquency: Empirical Testing of Seven Theories
Schoenthaler, SJ, PhD, Dept. of Sociology, Cal State University-Stanislaus, Vol. 7(2): 108-131, 1986

The findings in 1,150 juveniles confined to an institution revealed that the "children who were served orange juice in one study were significantly less likely to commit antisocial behavior than the juveniles who did not receive the orange juice." This is attributed to probable malnutrition of the juveniles.

Fishbein's work suggests that "diet can be an effective method of treating low blood sugar induced antisocial behavior."

EAT BETTER, LEARN BETTER
Appleton Central High School: A Case Study, *Wisconsin Briefs* from the Legislative Reference Bureau of the Wisconsin State Legislature, Brief 05-7, March 2005,

http://www.legis.state.wi.us/LRB/pubs/wb/05wb7.pdf)

Appleton Central High School, a charter school serving troubled students, implemented a health program focused on nutrition, exercise and psychology.

The Menu

The school worked with Natural Ovens Bakery to provide healthy breakfasts and lunches. They eliminated soda and snack vending machines and banned any outside food or drink. Bottled water was provided free to students. The new menu included only natural foods: fresh fruits and vegetables, lean meats and wholegrain baked goods. When students and faculty saw the positive effects, the rest of the Appleton Area School District adopted similar nutrition standards.

Physical Activity

The program promoted exercise by encouraging the use of pedometers to measure steps taken per day. Students "moved around" more even in some classroom settings. The school used a walking bus route as part of its activity program. The students show benefit from stress relief and psychological benefits of exercise as well.

Evaluation and Results

After one year, teachers and administrators said that the students learned better, behaved better and enjoyed school more. Serious problems such as dropouts, expulsions, drug use, weapons and suicide dropped to levels near zero. Students and faculty said they have gained knowledge that will stay with them for life.

What lies ahead is an increasing awareness that children with cognitive, mental and emotional problems have physical conditions. In fact, the physical diagnosis often emerges before the mental or emotional. This overlap of disorders is very curious and, in fact, makes a lot of sense.

The body and mind work together.

Overlap in Children – of Cognitive, Metabolic and Inflammatory Disorders

"Obesity and ADHD may represent different manifestations of a common environmental oversampling syndrome: a model for revealing mechanistic overlap among cognitive, metabolic, and inflammatory disorders", Bazara, KA, Yun, AJ, Lee, PY, et al, *Medical Hypotheses*, Volume 66, Issue 2:263-269 (2006)

ADHD is linked to a variety of disorders including obesity, insulin resistance, diabetes, hypertension, depression, psychosis, sleep apnea, inflammation, autism and schizophrenia.

Physical, Emotional and Behavioral Conditions Co-Exist
Blackman, JA. MD, MPH; Gurka, MJ, PhD, "Developmental and Behavioral Comorbidities of Asthma in Children", *Journal of Developmental & Behavioral Pediatrics*, 28(2):92-99, April 2007.

Children with asthma, especially severe asthma, are at high risk of developmental, emotional, and behavioral problems, such as ADHD, depression, anxiety and learning disabilities.

As you can see, the medical community finds out more each day about how physical symptoms and conditions effect our emotions, thoughts and cognitive abilities. What we eat can make or break this connection. The next several chapters will help you make these very important food choices for yourself and your family.

Chapter Two

FOOD POWER: Supporting a Growing Mind & Body

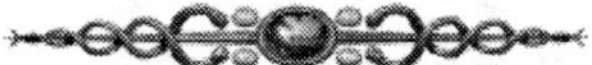

AAHH – the world of options. We are so fortunate to have mounds of selections in every food category imaginable. With these options, comes a need for information about what makes these foods different from one another – and most importantly, which are the healthiest for us.

The healthiest, most life-giving foods are the simplest – vegetables, fruits, legumes, nuts, seeds, lean animal products and good fats. We will reveal the best of the best in this chapter. Our focus is on what foods can support the growing bodies and brains of our children.

Protein: Foods & Snacks

Children require between 30-40 grams of protein daily. Every cell in the human body contains protein. It is a major part of the skin, muscles, organs, glands and most body fluids. The specific amount of protein is based on age, height and weight. Adults require 50-80 grams of protein per day.

Proteins are organic compounds which contain a chain of amino acids. Amino acids are the building blocks, and are also what is left after protein food is digested.

Children's bodies use amino acids to insure proper growth, development and repair of tissues. They are required in order to produce the brain chemicals or neurotransmitters and manufacture all hormones. Amino acids are necessary to catalyze or spark virtually all cellular activity!

Only 10 of the 20 amino acids are made in the human body. Consequently, amino acids are classified into two groups:

1. **Essential amino acids** cannot be made by the body and must be supplied by food. There are eight basic essential amino acids: phenylalanine, valine, threonine, tryptophan, isoleucine, methionine, leucine and lysine. Cysteine, tyrosine, histidine and arginine are generally regarded as essential, only for young, growing children, not adults. Sources of essential amino acids include eggs, poultry, fish, beef, milk, cheese, legumes, soy, nuts, seeds, sprouts, seaweed and algae products.

2. **Non-essential amino acids** are made by the body from the essential amino acids or normal breakdown of proteins. Their names are alanine, asparagine, aspartic acid, cysteine, glutamic acid, glutamine, glycine, proline, serine and tyrosine.

Protein-containing foods are considered either complete or incomplete:

1. **Complete proteins** contain all ten essential amino acids . They are found mostly in animal foods:
   - Meat
   - Fish
   - Poultry
   - Eggs
   - Milk
   - Milk products: yogurt & cheese

   Soybeans are the only plant protein considered to be a complete protein.
2. **Incomplete proteins** are missing one or more of the essential amino acids. Sources of incomplete protein include beans, peas, nuts, seeds and grains. A small amount of incomplete protein is also found in vegetables. To be incomplete is not bad; some foods are not meant to be complete proteins. Vegetables are one example. It just means incomplete protein foods must be combined with others, in order to become a complete protein.

Examples of food combinations that make complete proteins:

- Beans and rice (Legumes and rice)
- Almond butter on whole grain bread (Nuts and grains)
- Minestrone soup (Vegetables, whole grain pasta and beans)
- Yogurt with blueberries, walnuts and sunflower seeds (Fermented dairy, fruit, nuts, seeds)
- Rice or hemp protein powder with fruit juice and a capsule of blue green algae

Remember that foods high in amino acids, the building blocks of protein, can feed the neurotransmitters of the brain and help to balance blood sugar. It is important to choose protein foods that the child can digest easily. Proteins from vegetable sources are traditionally the easiest to digest and assimilate. Animal proteins, if lean, are also recommended, but may need some digestive support. This is why it is advised that a digestive enzyme is taken with a protein snack or meal --- so the child gets the benefit of the protein he or she has just eaten. The muscles and the brain need a steady stream of protein.

"Grab and Go" Proteins

These foods are suitable for the protein portion of a meal, or as a snack "on the run":

- slice of turkey, chicken, beef or other meat
- poached or scrambled egg
- all beef, organic hot dog
- vegetarian options: tofu hot dog, veggie burger, tempeh burger
- 2-3 oz. tuna salad or salmon salad
- 2-3 oz. chicken salad
- 2-3 oz. egg salad
- vegetarian option: "egg-less" tofu salad
- ¼ cup cottage cheese
- piece of string cheese
- organic yogurt with agave syrup or fruit
- 3-6 oz. organic goat, dairy, soy, almond, or rice milk
- whey, rice or hemp protein powder in rice, goat, almond or soy milk
- handful of raw sunflower seeds, pumpkin seeds, pine nuts
- handful of almonds (also seed and nut combo trail mixes)
- gluten-free beef jerky

CARBOHYDRATES: The Good, Not-So-Good & the Ugly

Do you have the "guts" to go against the grain?

The carbohydrates are the foods that the body most readily converts into energy! Sugar is the fuel derived from all carbohydrates and the quality of the sugar determines the quality of energy. The word starch is synonymous with carbohydrate. The carbohydrate foods are all grains, all breads, baked goods, pastas, and all fruits and vegetables.

The Good

The best carbohydrates are the fruits and vegetables. Ultimately, if we could eat only proteins and fruits and vegetables, with modest amounts of fats, we would all be better off. Peer pressure, the media, and our taste buds are the challenge though. Snack foods, party foods, holiday foods, and food we often crave fall into the carbohydrate category – the not-so-good-carbs. You will find in this chapter, ideas about making the switch to better carbs more do-able and enjoyable.

The Not-So-Good

If the carbohydrate (bread, pasta, baked good, and root vegetable) is highly refined, where the nutrients and fiber have been milled away, then the food actually saps energy from the body. It is best to avoid these foods and use them only occasionally.

This is why we suggest incorporating the unrefined grains in the whole form before they are milled into flour. Examples of this would be brown rice or oatmeal. Second best are the whole grains or flours used in the form of breads, cereals, and pastas. These should be used on a rotational basis, so you get a wide variety of nutrients, tastes, and textures. This type of carbohydrate is going be easier on blood sugar balance, moods, digestion, and energy levels than a totally refined product. The label of the product should read "whole" or "whole grain".

The Ugly: Wheat and Gluten

The over-abundance of wheat in our diets has caused many children to become sensitive to it. Traditional wheat allergies will cause mucous congestion, ear infections, itchy eyes, ears, nose and throat, and skin rashes. Luckily we have a whole world of alternatives -- beans, grains, nuts and seeds that can be eaten whole or milled into flour and used in baking.

The over-abundance of gluten is yet another issue. Gluten is the protein fraction found in all wheat, rye, barley, triticale, spelt, kamut and their derivatives. Derivatives include malt, grain starches, hydrolyzed vegetable/plant proteins, textured vegetable proteins, grain vinegars, soy sauce, grain alcohol, flavorings and the binders and fillers found in some vitamins and medications.

If you've ever handled it, you know how sticky it is – but that's what makes it work so well in breads, muffins, cookies, cakes, pizza, and so much more. Wheat has the highest gluten content of any grain. It is also one of the heartiest grains and one of the easiest to grow; therefore it is found in almost everything.

A gluten allergy or sensitivity is different from a wheat allergy, although they can co-exist. Gluten can devastate the mucous membranes of the body, most of all the digestive tract. It can cause diarrhea, constipation, gas, bloating, and cramping. Most of all, it can lead to "leaky gut syndrome", where undigested proteins slip through the intestinal lining into the bloodstream, wreaking havoc. Many children and adults diagnosed with ADD, ADHD, Autistic Spectrum Disorder, depression, insomnia, celiac disease, chronic fatigue syndrome, developmental delays, asthma, and allergies are susceptible to gluten in this way and must avoid the foods that contain it.[1]

The first step toward eliminating gluten is eliminating wheat in its many forms: Wheat - Its Various Forms and Hybrids: (all contain gluten)

- Whole wheat
- White wheat
- Durum wheat
- Semolina
- Spelt or Mir
- Kamut
- Bulgur
- Einkorn
- Couscous
- Kasha
- Graham flour
- Bran
- Wheat germ
- Farina

What can substitute for the wheat that is contained in many foods? Your answer lies in the following lists of many, varied grains:

Wheat-free grains that contain gluten (or gluten-like molecules):

- Rye
- Barley
- Oats (This is a borderline grain, as explained above.)

Wheat-free, gluten-free grains or starches:

- Amaranth
- Arrowroot
- Artichoke flour
- Brown rice
- Buckwheat
- Corn yellow/blue
- Fava flour
- Garbanzo flour
- Millet
- Nut flours
- Certified gluten-free oats
- Potato starch flour
- Quinoa
- Sorghum or milo
- Soy
- Tapioca flour
- Teff flour
- White rice

(An extensive list can be found in the *Substitutions Chapter 9*.)

The above grains, beans, and seeds are dried and milled into flour that can be used in baking. Pastas, cereals, breads, cookies, cakes, muffins, pancakes, and other baked goods can be made from flour. Some of the common brands names for these products are Arrowhead Mills, Ener-G, Hain, Shiloh Farms, Ancient Harvest, Pamela's, Pacific Bakery, Oasis Bakery, French

Meadows, and Food for Life. Your health food store or favorite online outlet has many choices waiting for you.

Below is a chart of the grains and their classes. Note that oats are in both the toxic or offensive column as well as the non-toxic. This is because new research points to oats as being non-toxic for gluten-sensitive individuals, however, some people are still sensitive to them. So, it is advised to avoid oats when eliminating all gluten products, and then carefully and with a watchful eye, add them back in after several months to see if they are something that can be handled.

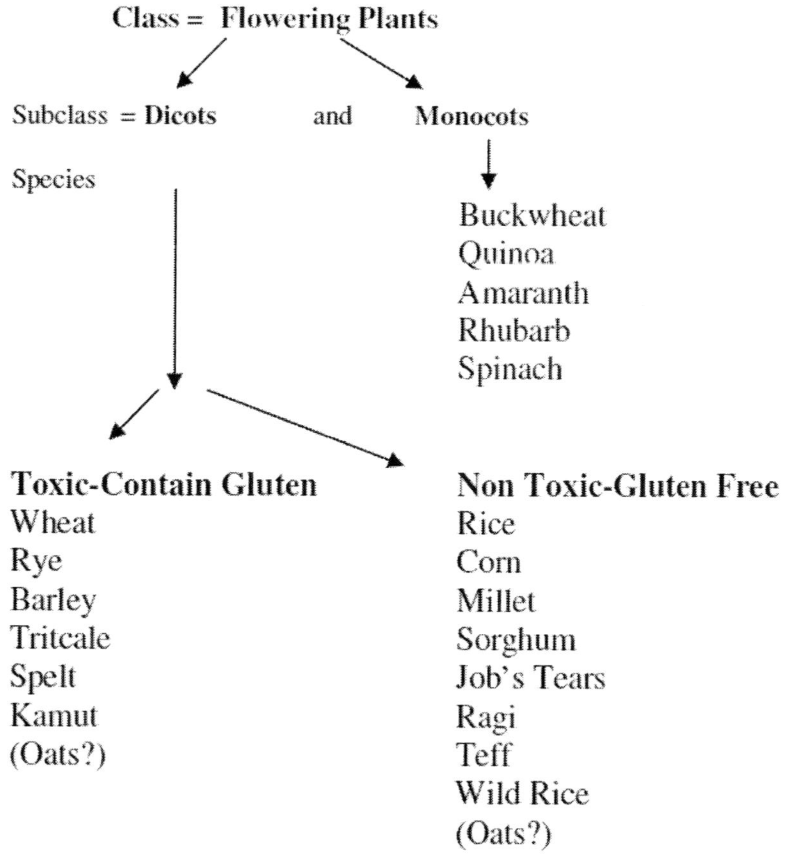

Note that all products in the wheat species column contain gluten. No other grain in the chart does. So from one standpoint, those are the only grains a gluten-sensitive individual should avoid.

There is a lot of controversy though, and misinformation in the field of gluten- containing grains. Understand though, that gluten is a protein component of wheat (***gliadin*** is the component) but not of any other grain. However, due to reactions that people have had over time, barley (containing ***hordein***) and rye (containing ***secalin***) have come to be known as gluten-containing. This is not exactly true because their protein components are different, but they are similar enough and cause the same symptoms, that all three grains are known to be off limits for people who are gluten sensitive or have celiac disease. (See C*hapter 11*)

Oats have long been considered as containing gluten, but officially the protein component of oats is ***avenin***. Recent research has let oats "off the hook" and they are now considered to be a safe food for most celiacs.

However, since oats are often produced and handled in places where they become "contaminated" with wheat, some people need to avoid them. It depends on how sensitive a person is. So the word in the celiac community is to generally avoid oats, but re-introduce it after a period of time to see if it causes any symptomatic changes. There are, however, certified gluten-free oats available from www.glutenfreeoats.com, Bob's Red Mill and www.creamhillestates.com.

The protein component of corn is called ***zein***; rice contains ***orzenin***. These proteins are not toxic to celiacs or those who are gluten-sensitive. Although corn does not contain gluten, it may be an allergy for some people.

Other issues with grains and flours:

Glycemic index: After all is said and done, there are other cautions about grains and flour foods that we must point out. Most importantly is that of "glycemic index". This is a way of classifying carbohydrates as to the effect they have on the blood glucose levels. All carbohydrates, grains and flour foods metabolize into sugar which is then available for energy. Whether that energy is strong and consistent, or highly fluctuating, depends on the glycemic index of that food. High-glycemic foods which cause energy imbalances should be minimized. Some high-glycemic, gluten-free grains are white rice flour, tapioca flour and potato flour. They elicit a high insulin response and are troublesome for people with sugar-handling problems. For children and teens with ADD, ADHD, autism, depression, mood disorders and PMS, it may be best to keep consumption of these foods to a minimum.

Fiber: Another issue with some gluten-free flours, especially the white ones, is that they are low in fiber. White rice, potato and tapioca flours are fairly refined. Care should be taken to keep the diet balanced and use these products minimally.

Cross-contamination: Cross-contamination is very prevalent in our commercial food industries. It would have to be, in our multi-tasking world. Wheat and gluten-containing crops are milled and processed under the same roof as gluten-free products. Sometimes they are grown near each other, stored together or prepared on the same surface. For sensitive people, this is critical, as they can react to the gluten-free product as if it contained gluten, due to "contamination". Bizarre, but true!

Let's Get the Fats Straight

It feels really good when you understand something that you usually shake your head about. Knowing fat facts can be very empowering for both you and your family. Remember that the brain is made of almost 60% fat. The fats you choose make a big impact. So many words are bantered about and you wonder ... what does this all really mean? So here we go --- **Fat Facts Made Easy**!

The words fats, oils, lipids, cholesterol and triglycerides have been used interchangeably. Here is what they really mean:

1. **Fat** – liquid or solid containing three free fatty acid molecules hooked to a glycerol molecule.

2. **Oil** – liquid fat.

3. **Lipid** – a general term that encompasses all types of fats and fatty acids.

4. **Cholesterol** – waxy, fatty substance found in animal foods, but also made in our bodies, in the liver. This a specific type of fat that is not made by plants. It has many important functions, including the manufacture of hormones. When it is oxidized, it becomes a health problem.

5. **Triglycerides** – a molecule of fat or oil, stored in the body's tissues or seeds of a plant.

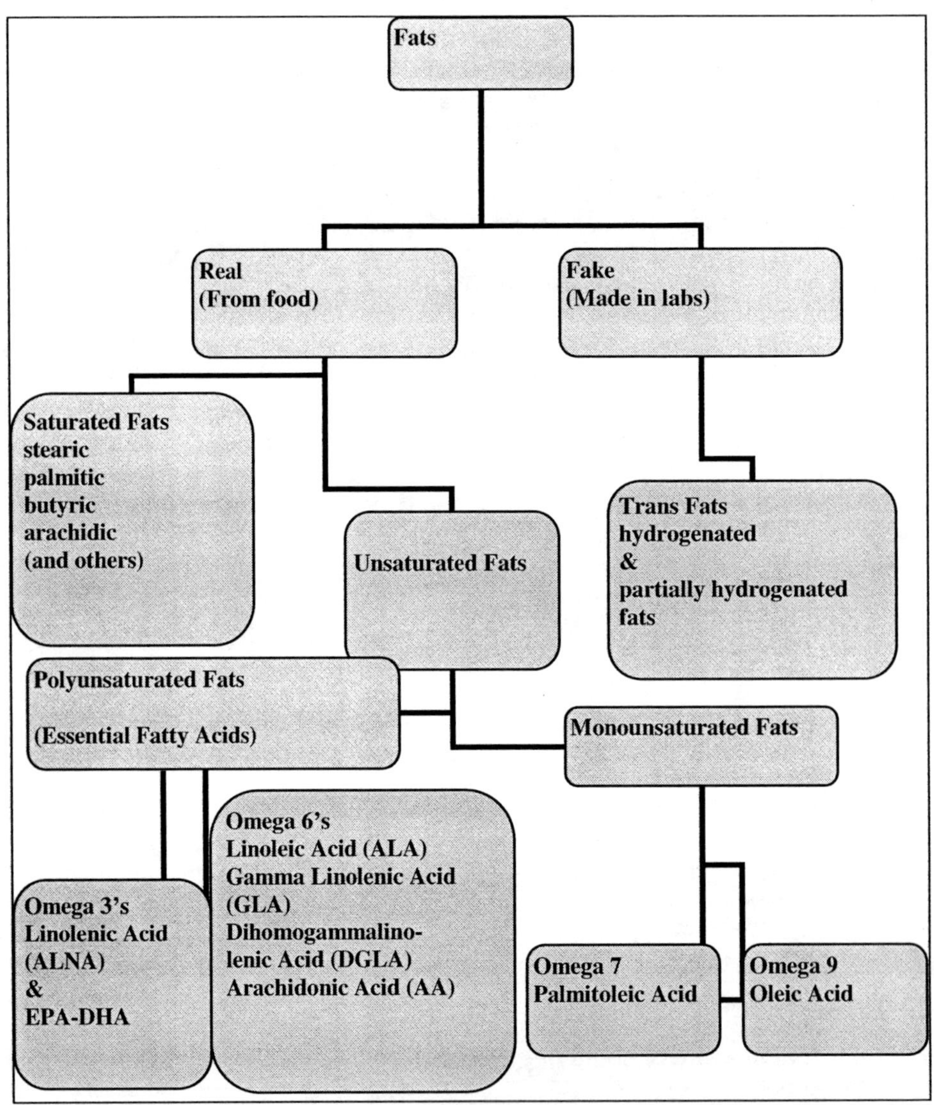

Choosing Between Saturated and Unsaturated Fats

The following information will help you choose the right fats for your child or ask your doctor the "right on" questions. There are two basic families of real fats: saturated and unsaturated. Both groups contain fats that have purpose or benefit for the body. They offer different qualities; for instance, the polyunsaturated fats are known to be helpful for parts of the body that have high activity, like the brain and eyes.

There is a group of fats that is not natural -- the trans fats. They start out as unsaturated fats, but are manipulated in a lab and the molecules are altered. They have no purpose or benefit for the body.

But they are prevalent in today's food supply, so we include them in the chart below:

Type of Fat	Main Source	Effect on Cholesterol Levels
Mono unsaturated	Olive oil, canola oil, peanut oil, olives, cashews, almonds, peanuts and most other nuts, avocados, canola seeds and oil	Lower LDL (bad cholesterol); raises HDL (good cholesterol)
Poly unsaturated	Fish, corn, soybean, safflower, and sunflower oils, cottonseed oil, tofu, pecans, hazelnuts, flax, hemp	Lower LDL and HDL, Lowers total cholesterol, contain Essential Fatty Acids (EFA's)
Saturated	Beef, pork, bacon, lard, egg yolks, coconut milk, palm, and palm kernel oils, whole milk, butter, cheese, cream and ice cream, chocolate, nut milk, cocoa butter, non dairy substitutes	Raise both LDL and HDL
Trans fats	Most commercial baked goods, most margarines, vegetable shortening; partially hydrogenated vegetable oil; many fast foods; deep-fried chips	Raise LDL (bad cholesterol); Lower HDL (good cholesterol) Cause inflammation Increase risk of diabetes

Important Distinctions

- The difference between saturated and unsaturated fats is that the unsaturated ones contain at least one double bond in their chain of atoms. Without going into a whole chemistry lesson, suffice it to say that the double bond causes certain instability within the chain of molecules, enabling them to become broken apart. They are then, easier to digest and become more fluid in the circulation.

- This is favorable, but is also why they are easily damaged by light, air, heat, water and time.
- Saturated fats, on the other hand, are hooked tightly together. This makes them harder to digest and causes them to clump in the body.[2]

Unsaturated Fats

The unsaturated fats are mostly found in products that are derived from plants, such as vegetable oils, nuts and seeds, and their oils. These fats have many benefits, not the least of which is improving blood cholesterol levels.

a) Monounsaturated fats are considered to be healthy because they not only lower the bad cholesterol, but they also help to increase the good cholesterol, whereas polyunsaturated fats lower both your bad cholesterol and good cholesterol. They also help keep the arteries supple.

Monosaturated fats include Omega 9's most known for being found in olive oil. The best type of olive oil is extra virgin, unheated. Omegas 9's are also found in almond, avocado and other nut oils.[3]

Recent research worth mentioning is about the Omega 7 oil from sea buckthorn or (Hippophae rhamnoides), a fruit from the sea. This oil has been used in Chinese and Tibetan medicine for more than twelve centuries. It is helpful for healing both the external as well as the internal skin – mucosal linings of the GI tract and urinary tract. The berries and seeds of sea buckthorn also deliver Omega 3, 6 and 9's.

b) Polyunsaturated fatty acids (PUFA's) are important because they contain omega-3 and omega-6 fatty acids, which are the essential fatty acids (EFAs). EFAs are important to good health and the overall well-being and growth of the human body. A deficiency in EFAs has been associated with depression, diabetes, cardiovascular disease, cancer and degenerative diseases such as multiple sclerosis. Omega-3's are found in oily fish, flax, hemp and soybean oils, as well as pumpkin seeds and walnuts. Omega-6's are found in unrefined safflower, corn and sunflower oils.

Saturated Fats

Saturated fats are found in all food fats and oils, especially hard fats such as animal fats and tropical oils. Specifically, they are found in meat, seafood (especially shellfish), poultry skin, egg yolks, coconut, palm and palm kernel oil. They are solid at room temperature.

Saturated fats raise total blood cholesterol more than dietary cholesterol because they increase both good and bad cholesterol. Though there is an increase in the good cholesterol, however, the net effect is a negative one. Therefore, saturated fats should be limited in the diet.

The prominent saturated fats are:

Stearic – found in beef, mutton, pork, cocoa butter

Palmitic – found in coconut, palm and palm kernel oil

Butyric – found in butter

Arachidic – found in peanuts.[4]

Other saturated fats are myristic (from palm, butter, and nutmeg), caprylic (from coconuts and breast milk) and lauric (from coconuts and palm kernel oil). They contain special immune protection properties and are found mostly in nutritional supplements as well as topical products and cosmetics.

Trans Fats

Trans fatty acids are contained in hydrogenated and partially hydrogenated fatty foods. They are produced via hydrogenation or heating of liquid vegetable oils such as corn and soy, in the presence of hydrogen. This is done to increase the shelf life of commercially prepared cookies, pies, cakes, margarine, shortening and fast foods.

Originally, it was thought that these fats were good replacements for saturated fat, but they were found to be devastating to our health, so they are now being banned in other countries. In fact, just recently, some fast food chains in the U.S. decided to eliminate trans fats from their menus.

Trans fats raise bad cholesterol and on top of that, decrease good cholesterol. They can also contribute to inflammation, implied as a cause of heart disease, stroke, diabetes and other chronic conditions. Obviously, trans fats should be greatly reduced or eliminated from your family's diet.

The Controversy over Coconut Oil

There have been many politically-driven, or should I say – greed-driven decisions in the food industry – probably forever. One such controversy has been over saturated fats, such as coconut oil. I think the decision was – "Move over coconut and palm oil and make way for the trans fats." And so we did and we are worse for it. Luckily, enough smart people realized what was going on and the trend now is to accept saturated fats for their health benefits – but only if they are high quality and unrefined.

Coconuts are 92% saturated fat, which often makes people avoid them. But all saturated fats are not created equal. 65% of the saturated fats found in coconut are what is called "medium chain." Medium chain fats have unique characteristics that set them apart from the other fats. For example, they do not require bile from the liver for digestion, so they are quickly absorbed and used by the body for quick energy. In this way, they resemble carbohydrates and are excellent for children.

Medium chain fats can be concentrated into a separate supplement called MCT oil. This oil is good for people with liver/gallbladder issues who need the energy from fat, but have trouble digesting it in food. Athletes also use this oil for quick energy. Medium chain fats protect the body from disease by disabling and killing bacteria, viruses, and parasites.

Sautéing with organic, unrefined coconut oil provides great flavor and texture to vegetables. It can also be added to smoothies and shakes. No fishy flavor or smell!

General Recommendations for Fat Intake

The bottom line is that we need to replace the bad fats (saturated and trans-fats) with high quality, organic and as-unrefined-as-possible good fats (mono- and polyunsaturated fats). However, it is also important to note that all fat, the good and the bad, contains the same number of calories.

Therefore, keep your fat intake to 20-30% of your total daily calorie intake.

The Essential Fatty Acids

Our children desperately need them!!! Low fat diets and fat-free foods go out the window! Essential fatty acids are vital for production of neurotransmitters, membranes of the neurons or brain cells and glial cells, and the very important double membrane of the blood brain barrier.

Here are other benefits of essential fatty acids:

- Fortify the brain: remember it is made of 60% fat
- Promote healthy nervous system
- Strengthen immune function and protection from infection
- Build bones
- Fortify healthy skin, hair, nails
- Improve eczema, psoriasis and acne
- Heal intestinal lining and inflammatory gut issues
- Balance other inflammatory issues – arthritis, fibromyalgia, allergies
- Lower risk of cardiovascular disease
- Enhance liver and gall bladder function
- Vital for adrenal, thyroid and sex hormone balance

Fatty Acid Deficiencies: What to Look for in Your Child

Many children have fatty acid deficiencies – mostly because there is either a predominance of bad or "fake" fats in their diet. The following symptoms are displayed in children with fatty acid deficiencies:

- Allergies
- "Alligator" or leathery skin
- Asthma
- Attention deficits
- Brittle, easily frayed nails
- "Chicken skin"
- Constipation
- Cracked skin on heels or fingertips
- Dandruff
- Dry eyes
- Dry skin
- Dry, unmanageable hair
- Excessive thirst
- Fatigue
- Frequent infections
- Frequent urination
- High cholesterol
- Hyperactivity
- Irritability or anxiety
- Leaky gut syndrome or malabsorption
- Learning disabilities
- Lowered immunity
- Obesity
- Patches of pale skin
- Poor growth
- Poor wound healing
- Soft nails

Fatty acids in general, are the major components of all fats and lipids. There are many different types. Some are good, some are not; some are essential and some are not. The body does produce some fatty acids, but not the essential ones.

Essential fatty acids **must** be taken in by the food we eat. **Essential means must have!** Our children's brains, nerves, hearts, livers and immune systems depend on them. And because fats are often difficult to digest, it may be helpful to take a digestive enzyme supplement along with the meal.

It is also important to remember how delicate essential fats are. They are easily damaged by light, air, heat, metals, water and time in storage. They should be pressed, filtered, packaged, stored and used with care. This means you should seek manufacturers who pay attention to their delicate nature. Suggested companies that oversee and take care of their oils are Premier Research, Udo's Choice (Flora Oils) and Spectrum Naturals.

Two Families of Essential Fatty Acids – Omega 6's and Omega 3's

Get ready for all the acronyms. There are two basic groups of essential fatty acids (EFA's) from the polyunsaturated group:

1. Omega 6, linoleic acid or LA
2. Omega 3, alpha linolenic acid, ALNA.

These two groups of EFA's and other general fatty acids in the body fall into two major families. Each family contains a separate set of fatty acids, which not only have different food sources, but also individual functions:

Omega 6 Family

Linoleic Acid (LA)

The fatty acids in the Omega 6 group are derived from food sources grown in warm climates. LA or linoleic acid is the main EFA in this group and is commonly found in seed oils.

Gamma Linolenic Acid (GLA)

Once in the body LA can make GLA or gamma linolenic acid. GLA is found almost exclusively in borage seeds, black currant seeds and evening primrose oil. GLA has great anti-inflammatory properties and helps with emotional balancing. It can be especially helpful for children with asthma and allergies.

Dihomogamma Linolenic Acid (DGLA)

This fatty acid is contained in mothers' milk and has great health benefits for immune, cardiovascular and kidney function.[5]

Arachidonic Acid (AA)

Arachidonic acid is also a member of the Omega 6 family. After a series of chemical changes, the body can manufacture it from linoleic acid. Arachidonic acid or AA is linked with the production of certain prostaglandins, hormone-like chemicals that in this case, cause pain and degenerative illnesses. When there is an abundance of AA in the body, this is what happens --- and it happens quite a bit nowadays, because we eat an excessive amount of Omega 6-containing foods.

The sources of arachidonic acid in food are: meat, poultry, dairy products, eggs and seafood. I'm not suggesting that we eliminate them, but balance them with the beneficial fatty acids, especially the Omega 3's. Many of these foods have a combination of Omega 3's and 6's.

Omega 6 Vegetable Oils

Omega 6 vegetable oils are a mixed bag. They are so prominent in our commercial food supply. Some of them are major culprits in the declining health of our lip-smacking, snacking, fast food society. Many of these oils are derived from seeds such as safflower, sunflower, sesame, and canola. The best omega 6-containing oil is organic olive oil, extra virgin and cold pressed.

Omega 3 Family

Alpha Linolenic Acid (ALNA)

Foods that contain ALNA are grown in cold weather climates. Flax seeds and oil are good examples. ALNA has anti-inflammatory and immune enhancing properties, as well as cognitive and cardiovascular-strengthening abilities. It is excellent for the digestive tract, skin and nervous system.

Vegetarian sources of ALNA such as flax oil, can convert to EPA and DHA in the body and that is good. The success of this conversion, however, depends on the efficiency of the liver and metabolic function of the individual. It is for some people, better to get the EPA and DHA from the source, rather than depend on the body to convert them.

Other excellent vegetarian sources of ALNA are hemp seeds and oil, pumpkin seed oil, soy bean oil, walnut oil, green leafy vegetables, acai palm fruit and freshwater blue green algae. Use the organic and unrefined versions.

Yes, sounds odd, but there are fatty acids in freshwater blue green algae. The best algal species for polyunsaturated fatty acids (PUFA) is Aphanizomenon flos-aquae (AFA). It is harvested in Klamath Lake, Oregon and contains about 50% PUFA's -- one reason it is known for enhancing the brain.

AFA Blue Green Algae: Good Source of Good Fats

"Favorable Effects of Blue-Green Algae Aphanizomenon flos-aquae on Rat Plasma Lipids," Kushak RI, Drapeau C, Van Cott EM, *JAMA*, vol. 2, No. 3, 2000, pp. 59-65.

Purpose-To investigate the effect of diets supplemented with algae on blood plasma fatty acids, cholesterol and triglycerides.

Results-Rats fed a diet free of polyunsaturated fatty acids (PUFA's) showed an absence of linolenic acid (LNA) in plasma. However, supplementation with algae resulted in the same level of LNA as controls, and increased levels of EPA DHA (eicosapentaenoic acid and docosahexaenoic acid), and a decreased level of arachidonic acid. (It is good that this fatty acid decreased.) Plasma cholesterol decreased between 25% and 54%, depending on the amount of algae eaten. Triglyceride levels also decreased.

Conclusion

Algae Aphanizomenon flos-aquae is a good source of PUFA and because of potential cholesterol-lowering properties, should be a valuable nutritional resource. (50% of lipids in AFA blue green algae are polyunsaturated fatty acids (PUFA's).[6,7]

EPA DHA (eicosapentaenoic acid and docosahexaenoic acid)

ALA goes through a series of changes in the body to produce EPA and finally DHA. These are important for the production of certain prostaglandins that enhance brain function in children and adults and development of brain activity for the fetus.

EPA and DHA are popularly known for being inherent in fish oils, such as wild salmon and cod. This is why salmon, salmon patties and cod liver oil are such great sources of brain nutrition for children with ADD/ADHD. The EPA and DHA support brain, eye, auditory and cardiovascular functions. DHA is one of the most abundant fatty acids in the fetal and infant brain.

Other EPA DHA sources are from high fat, cold water fish such as albacore tuna, sardines, anchovies, Atlantic halibut, pink and king salmon, krill (shrimp-like plankton), Pacific and Atlantic herring, Atlantic mackerel and lake trout. Oysters also contain a small amount of EPA and DHA.

Ratio of Omega 3's to Omega 6's

Our standard American diet does not offer many foods with the proper ratio of omega 3's to omega 6's. In fact the ratio is grossly distorted. Most people ingest somewhere between 1:10 and 1:20 omega 3's to omega 6's. The ideal ratio is however, 2:1, omega 3's to omega 6's.[8]

Without the proper ratio, many people, including children are predisposed to allergies and other immune problems, asthma, skin disorders, and inability to manufacture the proper membranes and neurotransmitters that effect balanced moods, emotions, behavior, focus and concentration. The proper ratio also promotes a healthy balance of cholesterol and triglycerides in the blood.

Sources of EFA's

Linoleic acid or LA (Omega 6)

Safflower oil
Sunflower oil
Flax seed oil
Pumpkin seed oil
Soybean oil
Walnut oil
Sesame oil
Navy beans (small amount)
Pinto beans (small amount)
Honey comb (beeswax)
Blue green algae

Linolenic acid or LNA (Omega 3)

Flax seeds and oil
Chia seeds and oil
Kukui or candlenut oil
Hemp seeds and oil
Pumpkin seed oil
Canola oil
Walnuts and walnut oil
Chestnuts
Hazelnuts
Dark green leafy vegs (sm amt)

Gamma linolenic acid or GLA (Omega 6)	**EPA & DHA (Omega 3)**
Borage oil	Wild salmon and salmon oil
Black currant seed oil	Cod and cod liver oil
Evening primrose oil	Trout
Mackerel	Sardines and anchovies
Brown and red algae	Krill oil (shrimp-like plankton)

What Interferes With EFA'S?

Essential fatty acids are very delicate and much care should be taken in preparation of the foods which contain them.

1. They are destroyed by foods that contain hydrogenated or partially hydrogenated oils such as margarine, crackers and chips.

2. Large quantities of sugar in our diets interfere with the body's use of EFA's.

3. If children are not eating whole foods, then it is likely their bodies are deficient in certain minerals and vitamins – the very cofactors necessary to help them process and use EFA's. The EFA's will not be absorbed.

4. Chemical pollutants in our food, water and air interfere with the absorption of EFA's. Lead, aluminum and cadmium are three that are very toxic and known to block EFA absorption.

5. Pervasive cooking methods, such as boiling, deep-frying and microwaving promote the destruction of EFA's in our children's bodies.

6. EFA's are perishable, deteriorating rapidly when exposed to light, air, heat and metals. Flax seed oil and hemp oil should be bought and stored in opaque containers to shield it from the light and refrigerated at all times.

It is easy to see how some children become deficient in essential fatty acids. To begin with, they are deficient in our food supply and then we destroy them with extreme-heat cooking methods. I strongly recommend that children receive liquid oil or capsule forms of various essential fatty acid supplements on a daily basis. I also suggest rotating different varieties in order to get the full spectrum of benefits.

The following studies indicate that Omega 3 and 6 fatty acids can help children with ADHD:

Omega 3's and 6's May Help ADHD
Sinn, N, PhD, Bryan, J, PhD, "Effect of Supplementation with Polyunsaturated Fatty Acids and Micronutrients on Learning and Behavior Problems Associated with Child ADHD", *Journal of Developmental & Behavioral Pediatrics*, 28(2):82-91, April 2007.

Strong positive effects of Omega 3 and Omega 6 fatty acids were found with ADHD children. They had improvement with inattention, impulsivity and hyperactivity.

Fish Oil Supplements Ease ADHD Symptoms
ABC News Online, June 21, 2006

Scientists at a university in Australia said that fish oil can be as effective at treating hyperactive children as conventional medicines such as Ritalin and Concerta, without the side effects.

When 130 children between the ages of 7 and 12 with ADHD were given fish oil and evening primrose oil capsules daily, behavior dramatically improved in 3 months. Also, after seven months, the children were less restless and had improved concentration and attention by one-third. These improvements continued after the study ended, which suggests the oils may have long-term effects.

Author's Comment: This is a mere example that nutrients can be very effective for brain function. The situation is not however, so black and white. Nutrients don't substitute for drugs; a well nourished balanced body, however can.

---

1. *Celiac Disease Foundation, Studio City, CA 818-990-2354, www.celiac.org*
2. *Erasmus, Udo, Fats that Heal, Fats That Kill, Burnaby, BC, Canada, 1996*
3. *IBID p.22*
4. *IBID p.23*
5. *IBID p.22*
6. *Bruno, Jeffrey, PhD., Edible Microalgae, A Review of Health Research, Center for Nutritional Psychology Press, 2001, P.25*
7. *"Favorable Effects of Blue-Green Algae Aphanizomenon flos-aquae on Rat Plasma Lipids," Kushak RI, Drapeau C, Van Cott EM Journal of American Nutraceutical Association, vol. 2, No. 3, pp. 59-65*
8. *http://www.udoerasmus.com*

Chapter Three

We Are What We Digest & Absorb

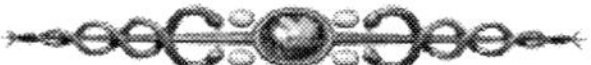

Food is power. It is our fuel. It produces brain and muscle energy, but it must be digested and absorbed in order to really power us. The digestive system, its organs, glands, enzymes and secretions break down foods into nutrients that our bodies can utilize. This is how we get the building blocks for bones, muscles and brain tissue; this is how we get nutrition; this is how we grow.

Much of our bodies' energy is utilized for the digestion and absorption of food. The brain requires fuel to do its job, and glucose from our food is that fuel. Effective digestion and absorption of nutrients into the bloodstream are imperative for brain function. It is easy to see the connection between the digestive tract and the brain when you realize this.

Experts say that 60-70 million Americans are affected by digestive disorders.[1] Many doctors and scientists believe that good health begins in the digestive tract. The American Cancer Society recognizes that a large number of cancers begin in the digestive tract. There are more digestive cancers than breast or prostate cancer.[2] This implies that a whole lot of people have preventable diseases – diseases of the digestive tract. And if you heal the digestive tract, there is a good chance the disease will not manifest. It makes sense when you think about it. If you don't have or are not absorbing the nutrients necessary to grow, repair and feed your organ systems, you can't thrive.

The majority of us have had a digestive problem in our lifetime. Some people have them every day, and know it. Others have them every day, and don't know it. Many parents don't know about the frequency and quality of their child's bowel movements. We haven't been taught that this is necessary information; nor have we been taught what to look for. Children can't always express what symptoms they have and the "poop" and "fart" topics usually bring about laughter, embarrassment or avoidance. Most digestive problems either go unnoticed or are accepted as normal. Common, they may be; normal, they are not.

First of all, everyone should have at least two full bowel movements per day, in one piece, about the size of a large banana. The color should be medium to dark brown. Frequency, size and consistency help to determine whether or not a person is fully digesting and absorbing his or her food. Proper elimination also helps expedite toxin release, which keeps the body detoxified or purified naturally. If toxins accumulate, fermentation, gas and infections may result, causing discomfort and leading to infections and degenerative diseases down the road. Yes, degenerative diseases can result from something that starts as a simple digestive imbalance. It is a chain reaction effect. Let's examine this further.

Digestive Problems

Digestion problems are many and varied. Common complaints are:

- gas and bloating – flatulence, distended belly
- stomach aches or cramping
- heartburn and acid reflux (child may clear the throat excessively)
- constipation – dry, small or infrequent stools (sometimes painful)
- diarrhea – loose, watery stools

A significant number of children have difficult, painful bowel movements. This is torturous for them and for their parents. Sometimes the problem stems from a control issue, causing intentional withholding of the bowel movement. It is a complex behavior and may involve a variety of emotional reactions.

Why children withhold BM's?

In a study in the *Journal of Pediatrics* in 2004, it was revealed that 78 percent of children that had difficulty with potty-training or withheld bowel movements were constipated. About 93 percent of the children who avoided using the potty had hard bowel movements. They had pain and discomfort. Doctors who ran this study recommended that parents give their children enough fluids and high fiber diets, including whole grains.[3]

Other problems concerning withholding BM's are:

- obtain sense of control
- experience embarrassment
- seek privacy
- think it's dirty
- avoid pain
- reacts to sounds of the bathroom – loudness or echoes
- experience anxiety – bathroom may be cold or maybe they feel awkward

Enhancing bowel function is imperative here and working with a behavioral specialist can be extremely helpful. Naturopathic doctors, homeopaths and holistic nutritionists will often have certain homeopathic remedies, super foods and digestive-enhancing products at their disposal that can help balance the emotional as well as the physical causes. Chiropractors and cranial sacral therapists can, through touch, hit the spot -- affecting a release that enables the child to breathe easy and let things flow. This usually succeeds with a holistic approach – body and mind working together.

Digestive conditions we know can result from impaired digestion.

The conditions listed below are medical diagnoses. They don't just fall out of the sky. They are degenerative and develop from the symptoms we have just discussed. It takes weeks, months and years for these conditions to develop, and as you'll see in the following section, it takes time for them to heal or reverse – but they can.

- Acid reflux
- Colitis
- Colon cancer
- Crohn's disease
- Diverticulosis, diverticulitis
- Hemorrhoids
- Infections – parasitic, yeast, bacterial, fungal
- Irritable Bowel Syndrome (IBS)

Conditions that we are <u>not</u> told can result from impaired digestion:

ADD/ADHD	Chronic Fatigue	Insomnia
Allergies	Depression	Mood swings
Asthma	Ear infections	Psoriasis
Bi-Polar Disorder	Eczema	Sinusitis
Bronchitis	Hyperactivity	Urticaria (hives)

Our attitudes and emotions are affected by pain, discomfort and malabsorption of nutrients that result from digestive problems. Therefore, attention deficits, fatigue, insomnia, irritability, depression, behavior and attitude problems in children may have their roots in the digestive tract.

Skin is Skin

The intestinal lining is considered the "internal skin". So, if there is irritation of the lining due to allergies or infection, then there may be problems with the "external skin". Common skin problems with children are eczema, psoriasis, rashes, itching and acne.

Infections of various types may be involved with digestive difficulties. These may be bacterial, yeast, fungal, viral or parasitic in nature. Children with a history of food allergies, ear infections, antibiotic use, sinusitis or sinus infections, asthma, bronchitis, thrush, colic, giardia, strep, staph or yeast infections should consider getting a specialized gastro-intestinal pathogen screening or specialized stool test. After all, the gastro-intestinal tract houses the largest part of our immune system.[4] You can discover vital information about your digestive and your immune health by doing this test.

Your health practitioner can provide you with the home-collection test kit for the stool and saliva samples. You send the test kit to the appropriate specialty laboratory, such as Diagnos-Techs Laboratory or Genova Laboratory. (See *Resources* in back of book.) Stool pathogen screening is also recommended for children in families with pets, children who attend daycare, and those who frequently eat school meals.

Another specialty lab, Entero Lab, offers stool testing for food sensitivities, especially for specific gluten sensitivity and intestinal illnesses. They also offer a genetic test for gluten with a simple swab of saliva.

The Dynamic Duo

The word is out! Our bodies and our brains have a very dynamic and intricate connection. Together, they make ... us. And their connecting link is the intestinal tract. It not only turns our food into fuel, but also is a crucial chemical factory for our thoughts and emotions. Below is a synopsis of the New York Times article, revealing that the "body has 2 brains".

"The Gut-Brain Highway: A 2-Way Street"
Blakeslee, Sandra, *New York Times*, January 23, 1996
"Complex and Hidden Brain in the Gut Makes Cramps, Butterflies and Valium": The body has 2 brains – one in the head and the other in the intestines or "the gut".

- When the brain "gets upset", so does the nervous system in the intestines, and vice versa.
- About 95% of the brain chemical, serotonin is manufactured in the intestinal tract.
- The brain chemicals, serotonin, dopamine, histamine, nitric oxide, enkephalins, and norepinephrine are found in the intestines.
- This is called the "enteric nervous system" and its neuro-chemicals communicate with those in the brain.

- Dr. Michael Gershon, professor at Columbia Presbyterian Medical Center in New York, says that the brain in the gut effects both happiness and misery. Thus, we hear the expressions: "gut feelings" and "butterflies in my stomach".

It is easy to understand the importance of maintaining an efficient digestive tract when you consider that brain chemical or neurotransmitter production is seated in the intestines as well as the brain.[5]

Remember, no one thinks straight when his mind is focused on the toilet!

The primary food habits associated with digestive problems are:

1. **Overeating** - You can't break down and assimilate food properly if you bombard the intestines with too much food or frequent eating.
2. **Eating too many concentrated foods** - Certain foods such as tomato sauces and salsa can contribute to an acidic digestive system, which may inactivate enzymes. Heavy, concentrated fats or proteins have slow transit times in the bowel and can inhibit digestion and absorption of foods with quicker transit times.
3. **Quality of the food you eat** - Refined food and processed foods are not only empty, but dead and toxic, causing the body to work harder to digest and detoxify them. They are also depleted of fiber, and don't move through the digestive tract very efficiently. Enzyme-depleted food draws on the body's natural resources for digestion. You can only rob your nutritional bank for so long before it is drained of the nutrients and enzymes you need for digestion, absorption and elimination.
4. **Late night eating** - Digestion, metabolism and sleep may all be affected adversely if we eat a meal too close to bedtime. The more tired a body is, the more sluggish the digestion will be. Try to eat at least 3 hours before sleep time. Some kids like to have a little something before bed. Make sure it is a whole food choice, like almond butter on a whole grain cracker or a handful of raw trail mix.
5. **Eating fast** - Eating too quickly and not chewing enough can cause incomplete digestion, hyper-acidity and difficult elimination. Remember that digestion begins in the mouth with the enzymes secreted in our saliva, and your food must mix with the saliva for enhanced digestion.
6. **"Emotional eating"** - Ingesting food when you are angry or tense can activate the "fight or flight" mechanism which inhibits normal digestive

activities. When we are depressed, frustrated or angry, we often reach for comfort foods with addictive qualities, such as caffeine and sugar.

7. **Eating offending foods** – Foods such as coffee, citrus fruits and juice, cooked tomato products (including pizza), fast food and fried food, shellfish and pork, onions and garlic, spicy food, carbonated drinks, wine, beer and hard alcohol can contribute to acid reflux, constipation, diarrhea, gas and bloating. In addition, any foods to which a child is allergic or sensitive can disrupt digestive processes.
8. **Food combining**: Certain foods are processed at different rates in the GI tract and some people benefit from certain food combinations.

   - Fruit is digested and absorbed much more quickly than any other food, therefore, it should be eaten separately. Combining it with other food causes fermentation in the intestines and can result in gas and bowel problems.
   - Carbohydrates and proteins (especially animal proteins) should not be combined in the same meal. They each utilize specific enzymes and are processed at different rates, putting stress on the digestive system. This saps energy.

Strict adherence to the above "rules" may be more important for some people than others. Adapting to these principles will help to improve mild to extreme digestive upsets. The consequence of a poorly functioning digestive system is malnourishment -- from lack of nutrients, not lack of food.

The quality and types of foods, diets and eating habits can contribute to digestive problems. Even infant formulas can be a culprit, and for that matter, so can mother's milk. It can start from day one, or develop over time. Let's look at how digestive problems begin.

Digestive problems are rooted in these areas:

1. **Dehydration** – This can result from low water intake, high excretion of fluids, and mineral or electrolyte deficiency.
2. **Vitamin and mineral depleted diet** – Refined food is depleted of nutrients and causes the body to work harder to digest it.
3. **Lack of good bacteria** in the small and large intestines is often caused by use of prescription medications, especially antibiotics. They deplete the good bacteria, killing the good and bad bacteria indiscriminately.
4. **Low output of digestive enzymes** from the pancreas can be caused by overeating processed foods that are enzyme-depleted. Over time, this uses up the body's natural enzyme resources.

5. **Low hydrochloric acid** in the stomach results in improper digestion of the proteins and amino acids that are necessary for brain activity, balanced energy and metabolism. This can contribute to acid reflux, esophageal regurgitation (GERD), raspy voice, or excessive clearing of the throat.
6. **Low bile production or availability** – Bile, produced by the liver and stored in the gall bladder is necessary for proper digestion, especially of fats. If a child has light colored (tan) stools, excessive gas, bloating, stomach aches or diarrhea, a bile deficiency may be indicated. This can cause fatty acid deficiency and inability to digest fried foods, animal products, creamy foods, oils and spices. Food allergies may also be prominent.
7. **pH imbalance** (acid/alkaline balance) – Certain parts of the GI tract are supposed to be alkaline and other parts, acidic. There is a good reason for this -- so that all types of foods can be digested. And there is quite a variety. Also certain digestive enzymes, bile and stomach acid require varied and specific pH levels in order to be sufficiently produced.
8. **Slow peristalsis** or muscular movement of food along the intestines can be caused by depleted enzymes, low nutrient intake, vitamin C deficiency or **fiber deficiency**. This can lead to constipation, malabsorption or fatigue.
9. **Essential fatty acid deficiency** can cause dry stools and an easily damaged intestinal lining.
10. **Vaccine damage** – Toxic metals in some vaccines can damage the intestinal lining. Also live cultures in vaccines can disturb the microbial balance of the gut, and the ratio of good bacteria and bad bacteria may be disrupted.
11. **GI tract infections** - Intestinal and bowel infections may be responsible for compromised digestion. Poor absorption, nutritional deficiencies, toxicity, active and/or chronic illness and degenerative disease may result. Pathogens are everywhere: yeast, Candida, fungus, staph, strep, and parasites. They can contribute to nutritional deficiencies, produce toxins, and lead to chronic illness.

Most of all, infections lead to malabsorption of nutrients and this is devastating for the brain and the metabolism. The body is “runnin’ on empty” and draws on its resources, stored macronutrients and micronutrients. In growing children, this can disrupt their development and cognitive function. Sleep and ability to handle stress are often affected because infections are stressful for the body and require the stress hormonal system to mediate. The consequences of this may be hidden or may be blatant. The child could have insomnia, hyperactivity, unexplained fears.

There are entire books written on the topic of how to improve digestion, absorption and elimination. We have an overview here, but this topic is very far-reaching. Like an octopus, the digestive system is connected to so many things – growth, weight, emotions, mental function, energy, sleep and the immune system. Of equal importance are the solutions that follow.

Solutions: The 4 - R Program

Because of the far-reaching effects of GI function on health, and because so many medical conditions are recognized as having a gastrointestinal component, the 4-R Program has been developed as a method of treatment. Many health professionals and patients favor this protocol because it is tried and true. It's been used for centuries. Put simply – it works. In brief, the 4 R's of the 4-R Program are:

1. **REMOVE**
2. **REPLACE**
3. **RE-INOCULATE**
4. **REPAIR**

1. REMOVE harmful foods, toxins, pathogenic organisms. This phase involves the removal of substances that may be contributing to the problem; it has several components: a) dietary, b) toxin removal and c) pathogen removal.

a. The dietary component involves an elimination diet or the removal of certain foods thought to be reactive. These foods may be allergens or intolerances. If you don't already know which foods to avoid, consult with a food allergy expert to get the proper testing. A good place to start is with the foods listed in the Allergy section of this book.

b. The "Remove" phase also involves reducing the "total load" of toxins. This includes dietary changes to eliminate the intake of food additives in prepared and processed foods, lifestyle changes to reduce/eliminate smoking, caffeine and alcohol, and reduction of toxic exposure from medications, household products, dental materials and other environmental toxins.

c. Another first step in restoring proper functioning of the gastrointestinal tract is to remove abnormal and potentially harmful organisms. A certain amount of harmful or pathogenic organisms is common – part of the balance of nature. However, if the population becomes overgrown, then we have an imbalance: an infection, pain, inflammation or damage to the intestinal tract. These pathogens are bacteria, parasites, yeast commonly known as "Candida", fungus and mold. Toxic metals such as lead and mercury may also be removed in this process.

- Drinking the appropriate amount of fresh, pure water is a main component of the removal process.
- Natural nutritional supplements such as grapefruit seed extract, artemesia annua, bentonite clay, oil of oregano, wormseed oil or black walnut oil may be used in this initial step.
- A gentle, warm-water enema with a capsule of acidophilus or colostrum can be helpful in the elimination process as well.
- Check with your health care practitioner on the appropriateness and frequency of use of the above remedies and techniques.

2. REPLACE digestive enzymes and stomach acid. The goal of the "replace" phase is to supply the GI tract with the elements required for proper digestion, such as hydrochloric acid and the pancreatic enzymes that may have become deficient. This can largely be attributed to the lack of enzymes in our food supply. With most cooking processes, especially microwaving and the processing of most of our grocery items, our food no longer has life quality. The enzymes are gone. This puts an added burden on our digestive tracts to produce more enzymes.

Therefore, it is imperative that most people, even those without apparent digestive symptoms, take digestive enzymes by capsule. Popular herbs and plants with digestive enzyme qualities are ginger, pineapple (bromelain) and papaya (papain). Another digestive "product" that may need to be replaced is hydrochloric acid, produced by the stomach. Some enzyme products contain hydrochloric acid (HCL) or additional stomach support nutrients such as vitamin B12 and glutamic acid.

Replacing proper functioning of enzymes in the digestive tract may help reduce allergic and inflammatory reactions caused by undigested food molecules.

Digestive Enzymes

Start your child with digestive enzymes that are plant-derived, containing all the necessary enzymes to help the body digest proteins, carbohydrates, fats, lactose (milk sugar) and cellulose (fiber). These enzymes are called protease, amylase, lipase, lactase and cellulase, respectively. Look for these listed on the label.

A "multiple" enzyme product with these components is optimal as it will help replenish the body with enzymes necessary for proper digestion and absorption of food. Remember, much of our food today is over-processed and over-heated, therefore, enzyme-depleted.

Think of enzymes as the keys that unlock the nutrients in the food. Without them, the nutrients remain locked up, not absorbable, and are wasted or eliminated.

Another point about digestive enzymes is that they can get into the bloodstream and actually work on and "digest" antibodies that cause allergic reactions and inflammation. For this purpose, it is best to try a digestive enzyme between meals, on an empty stomach. This will enable the enzymes to work on the protein debris in the blood, from viruses, bacteria and yeast, as well as antibodies.

3. RE-INOCULATE with prebiotics and probiotics - The goal of the "re-inoculate" phase is to restore to normal the bacterial flora of the GI tract. This has two effects. The first is to restore the normal "good" bacterial functioning in the digestive process. The second is to reverse the overproduction of harmful and inflammatory substances being produced by the abnormal "bad" bacteria that are present. The "re-inoculation" phase involves reintroducing not only the normal GI flora, but also the nutrients or "partners" they require for proper metabolic function. These are called "prebiotics", such as fructo-oligosaccharides (FOS). Both prebiotics and probiotics are available in capsule or powder form and often together.

Probiotics such as acidophilus and bifidus:

- Are beneficial bacteria that the body needs in the small and large intestine respectively, in order to create a proper acid/alkaline environment.
- Enhance the body's ability to absorb food and nutrients more efficiently.[6]
- Help eliminate gas, bloating, indigestion, poor assimilation of nutrients, poor and inconsistent bowel function
- Assist in the manufacture of vitamins B1, B6, B12, and folic acid.
- Help the body to stave off harmful bacteria that occur from taking antibiotics, other prescription medications, the birth control pill, drinking tap water, eating white sugar and white flour products.
- Manufacture the body's own antibiotics in the gut.

Re-populating the intestines with the acidophilus and bifidus is often imperative, especially with ADD and ADHD children who have a history of ear infections, respiratory problems, sinus infections, asthma, bowel problems or skin problems – particularly the children who have had antibiotic treatments.

Remember that we have 5-15 pounds of good bacteria in our intestines, about 400 different species! When gathered together, this would be about the size of the liver. These bacteria, though dispersed throughout the GI tract, function as an organ. This "organ" is nourished and revitalized with the "probiotic" supplements that restore the population of the good bacteria, and food is absorbed more efficiently. The child is better nourished; the body and brain become more balanced and vibrant.

Acidophilus produces lactase, the enzyme that aids in the digestion of milk sugars. Dairy eaters should definitely use acidophilus. It also produces lactic acid, which helps to balance the acid and alkaline levels in the intestines.[7] Acidophilus seems to have the ability to help lower high cholesterol levels and help to "unclog" the microvilli; little hair like structures that assist in moving food through the intestinal wall. Unclogging them, improves the absorption process and allows the lining of the intestines to heal and be fortified. This is very important for those with food allergies, especially wheat and gluten. Acidophilus also helps peristalsis, the movement of food through the GI tract.

Bifidus produces lactic acid as well. It also manufactures acetic acid, vitamin B12 and vitamin K. It is the predominant bacteria in the intestines of breast-fed infants. Factors in the breast milk encourage its growth. It is the most important friendly bacteria for infants.

Bifidus remains more abundant in healthy children and adults, than acidophilus. It also secretes substances that inhibit the growth of unfriendly bacteria, as well as Candida or yeast.

I'm sure some of you are asking the question, "Can we get the acidophilus and bifidus from yogurt?" The answer is, "Yes, if you make your own." It's easy to do, once you set up a system for it, and can be a reliable source of probiotics. If you choose to buy commercial yogurts, however, there is quite a range of quality available. Most of the yogurts from grocery stores do not contain "live" good bacteria.

If they do, the bacteria are Lactobacillus burgaricus and Streptococcus thermophilus and these are of little benefit, as they only live for a brief period in the intestinal tract. So, you do not find acidophilus and bifidus in most commercial yogurts. Additionally, many brands contain sugar, artificial sweeteners, or food colorings and preservatives.

As a parent, it is difficult to know what products to choose for your child. One suggestion is to log onto www.simplexityhealth.com and read about digestive enzymes, acidophilus and bifidus. There is a multitude of information on this website and if you place an order they will guide you toward people who can advise you further.

4. **REPAIRING** the intestinal lining and potential “leakage” is the last phase of the 4-R Program. The goal of this phase is the healing of the gastrointestinal tissue, which involves supplying the GI tract with the components needed for cellular repair and function. The lining of the intestinal tract requires restorative work after damage has taken place and possible “gut leakage” has occurred. (See section on Leaky Gut Syndrome). Subtle damage ranging to the most extreme can be repaired with a variety of natural products: amino acids such as glutamine and n-acetyl-glucosamine, zinc, calcium, vitamin A, vitamin C, DGL or deglycyrrhized licorice, aloe vera and fatty acids. Repairing the GI tract is also important because it houses the largest part of our bodies' immune system.[8] A strong formidable intestinal tract will help keep microorganisms at bay, as well as future digestive and other health problems from occurring.

4 R's Conclusion: When most people follow the system of “the 4R's”, symptoms and conditions concerning the digestive tract can be eradicated or reversed. Many parents don't realize that their children need these digestive products. It takes detective work and knowing what to look for, to really find out, because digestive problems may be very subtle.

I contend that parents can handle helping children through this digestive healing process. It helps enormously, however, to consult with your health practitioner before starting a gut-healing program, because he or she is a specialist in this area. Direction and focus are what your health practitioner can offer, as well as experience with gut healing products. When you see the cause and effect while being guided, you will gain tremendous insight and confidence. At a point, you will know when you are ready to make your own decisions. What an accomplishment that will be!

High Fiber Foods

High fiber foods enhance digestive and bowel function. The fruits listed are best raw and the vegetables are best raw or lightly steamed. If any of these foods are on your "avoid" list, please do so.

1. Baked potato with skin
2. Bran cereals: Oat bran, wheat bran, rice bran
3. Whole grains: Hot and cold cereals, whole grain breads and pastas (brown rice, whole wheat, buckwheat, amaranth, quinoa, etc.) Refined grains have minimal fiber content.

4. Dried beans, peas and other legumes, including baked beans, kidney beans, split peas, garbanzos, pintos, black beans
5. Fresh and frozen lima beans
6. Green beans or French beans
7. Fresh and frozen green peas
8. Brussels sprouts
9. Broccoli
10. Dark green, leafy vegetables: spinach, beet greens, kale, Swiss chard
11. Cabbage – steamed, raw, cole slaw
12. Steamed artichokes - Scraping the leaves with your teeth provides your body with great fibrous material.
13. Carrots
14. Fresh or frozen sweet corn: on or off the cob
15. Dried fruit: figs, apricots and dates
16. Fresh or frozen berries: raspberries, strawberries, blue or blackberries
17. Organic plums, pears, and apples -- because the skin is edible
18. Raisins and prunes
19. Cherries and grapes
20. Bananas
21. Coconut (fresh or dried, not processed)
22. Raw nuts: almonds, Brazil nuts, walnuts

The Grass is Greener When it's Watered!

Don't let water get lost in the sauce! We have so many other beverages that are popular and we tend to forget that it's not just liquids that we need but --- pure, fresh water. Many kids drink milk, soda, energy drinks, fruit juices and fruit punches, and we fail to realize that these are FOODS! Because of their sugar, fat or protein content, the body must activate digestion in order to utilize them.

Water on the other hand is a digestive aid. It is the medium with which we digest, dissolve, absorb, assimilate and transport nutrients throughout the body. Remember, the body is roughly composed of 25 percent solid matter and 75 percent water. Brain tissue is composed of 74 percent water and the blood is 83 percent water. This is key to good quality of life.

Water is necessary for numerous metabolic functions:

- Digestion of food
- Transport of food to the tissues
- Elimination of body wastes
- Circulation of body fluids (lymph and blood)

- Lubrication of joints and internal organs
- Passage of substances between the cells and blood vessels
- Regulation of body temperature
- Making dissolved minerals available to the body tissues

There is a fascinating book written on the topic of healing with water, called *The Body's Many Cries for Water*. The author, Dr. Batmanghelidj, was a medical doctor who, as a political prisoner in Iran, researched about the medicinal value of water. He later published a report in the *Journal of Clinical Gastroenterology*, in June of 1983.[9] His revelations range from eliminating headaches with water to normalizing blood pressure, to healing asthma and eczema.

The premise, upon which his book is based, is that many of us are dehydrated and don't know it. Either we're:

1. Not drinking enough water
2. The water is not absorbing into the cells, or
3. We have mineral deficiencies causing dehydration.

For many children and teenagers, water is an after-thought. First on their list is usually a cola, energy drink, mocha or iced tea. Kids are taking in more caffeine now than ever, and from this they become dehydrated. Water is the <u>only</u> liquid that hydrates or re-hydrates. Let's examine the effects this might have.

Symptoms of Dehydration

- Anxiety and depression
- Difficulty losing weight
- Digestive problems
- Dry lips and mouth
- Dry, itchy skin
- Excess body fat
- Headaches or migraines
- High blood pressure
- Kidney and bladder problems
- Lack of energy
- Muscle soreness
- Persistent constipation
- Poor muscle tone and size
- Rapid heart beat
- Short term memory loss
- Poor focus or concentration
- Water retention problems
- Wrinkling and poor skin tone

Many children with allergies, asthma, skin problems, constipation, stomach aches, arthritis, headaches and hyperactivity are actually dehydrated. **You can drink a lot of liquids and still be dehydrated,** especially if the liquids are sweet, as in fruit juices and sodas. These children may or may not be thirsty, but they are still dehydrated.

Dark, concentrated urine in small amounts, dry mouth, chapped lips, eczema, breathing problems and excessive thirst are all signs of dehydration in your child. Healthy urine is usually pale and yellow, and frequency of output should be about every two to four hours.

What Kind of Water is the Best?

Quality of the water is very important. Remember that the body thrives on food, air and water ---- so we'd better give it the good stuff. Standards for taste, odor and appearance are not uniform. Various chemicals including fluoride and chlorine are now mandatory in some water systems and have been found to have highly toxic side effects.

By all means, avoid tap water, unless you know for sure that it is pure. About 70 percent of the water in the U.S. is chlorinated and 50 percent is fluoridated. Chlorine has been linked to bladder cancer and reproductive problems and fluoride is toxic to the bones. Also, according to a survey conducted by the Environmental Working Group, 260 contaminants were found in tap water in 42 states in the US. These include industrial toxins, PCB's, pharmaceutical products, metals such as arsenic and other inorganic contaminants. Though these toxins were found at levels below the maximum safety standards, the cumulative effect, especially, over many years is unknown.[10]

Understanding Types of Water

About 25 percent of bottled water is purified and comes from municipal water sources. Commercial examples are the Aquafina and Dasani brands; 75 percent of bottled water is actually from underground sources, such as rivers, lakes, springs and artesian wells.

Artesian Water is bottled from a well that taps a confined aquifer (a water-bearing underground layer of rock or sand) in which the water level stands at some height above the top of the aquifer. No pump is needed to retrieve this water.

Spring Water comes from an underground formation from which water flows naturally to the earth's surface. It must be collected only at the spring or through a borehole tapping the underground formation feeding the spring.

Mineral Water naturally contains at least 250 parts per million total dissolved solids (TDS). This is the main difference between mineral water and spring water. It has to contain more minerals, such as calcium, magnesium and trace minerals in order to be called mineral water. Because of the high mineral content, the taste is stronger.

Purified Water has many synonyms. It has been produced by distillation, deionization, reverse osmosis or other suitable processes. Purified water may also be referred to as "de-mineralized water." It usually originates from municipal sources and may also be labeled “drinking water”. This water is not a good source of minerals.

Distilled Water is evaporated, then re-collected. The water is clean, but it contains no minerals. Avoid using too much distilled water because it contains no minerals and is, in effect, “dead”. It draws minerals and toxins out of the body and for this reason, is useful during periods of cleansing or fasting, but it is not recommended for daily use as your only water.

Sparkling Water contains the same amount of carbon dioxide that it had at emergence from the source. So it starts out as spring water and the CO2 or carbon dioxide may be removed and then replenished after treatment.

Specialty Waters are bubbling around us. Bottled water is a huge industry, so there are many kinds. It is best to avoid flavored water, which contains artificial sweeteners and other chemicals. There are other specialty waters, critically acclaimed for high absorbability. The water is organized into specific molecular structures. Some terms for these are Pentahydrate, micro-clustered or structured water. New studies are now emerging, revealing that some of these waters hydrate the cells at a very deep level, far beyond most commercial bottled waters.

All in all, one of the best choices is natural spring water because it collects minerals and good microorganisms as it rises up out of the ground. If you can buy it in glass bottles, that is the best. But it is rare.

Storing Water

Now – about plastic bottles. This is a most unfortunate situation. The majority of plastic water bottles have the potential of leaching toxins into the water. Even if the water itself is pure, a plastic container may leak chemicals such as phthalates, Bisphenol A or antimony into the bottled water. Storage in cool and dark places helps reduce leaching of these chemicals.

There is controversy about which plastic is best. Look for the number in the triangle on the bottom of the bottle; these are the plastic resin codes. Many say “1”. Some say “7” or a variety of other numbers. The #1’s are generally regarded to be the safest; however, there are problems with all the plastic options.

Plastics to Avoid (Look for the number inside the triangle at the bottom of the bottle.)

- #3 Polyvinyl Chloride (PVC) commonly contains di-2-ehtylhexyl phthalate (DEHP), an endocrine disruptor and probable human carcinogen, as a softener.
- #6 Polystyrene (PS) may leach styrene, a possible endocrine disruptor and human carcinogen, into water and food.
- #7 Polycarbonate contains the hormone disruptor bisphenol-A, which can leach out as bottles age, are heated or exposed to acidic solutions. Unfortunately, #7 is used in most baby bottles, five-gallon water jugs and in many reusable sports bottles.

Better Plastics

- #1 polyethylene terephthalate (PET or PETE), the most common and easily recycled plastic for bottled water and soft drinks, has also been considered the most safe. However, one 2003 Italian study found that the amount of DEHP in bottled spring water increased after 9 months of storage in a PET bottle. Also antimony trioxide is used as a catalyst in the manufacture of PET and can leach out of the plastic into the water, if the bottle gets too hot or the water is stored for over six months.[11]
- #'s 2, 4, and 5 are secondary options for plastic bottle use.

Better Baby Bottles: Choose tempered glass or opaque plastic made of polypropylene (#5) or polyethylene (#1), which do not contain bisphenol-A.

Safety Tips for Using Plastic Bottles:

- Catch a whiff. Take a taste. If you can smell or taste plastic, don't drink it.
- Keep bottled water away from heat, as it causes metals and other chemicals to leach into the water.
- Use bottled water quickly, as storing it may cause leaching from the plastic. Don't store over six months.
- Most bottles are not re-usable, due to more bacterial growth and chemical leaching.
- Choose strong, reusable containers or thermoses with stainless steel or ceramic interiors. This is especially important for hot or acidic liquids.

- Use wide mouth Nalgene bottles made from safer plastic, from www.campmor.com. They are easily cleaned and don't accumulate as much bacteria.
- We highly recommended transferring your water from plastic to a stainless steel or a glass container.

You are going to have more control over the quality of water your family drinks, if you filter it yourself. Reverse osmosis is a good choice for filtration and as long as you regularly change the filters, you'll have reliable water. You can filter your well water or your municipal water. Many unwanted substances and contaminants are removed during this process, including most of the fluoride. About 75 percent of the minerals are also extracted, so a smart thing to do is to add a pinch of sea salt or your favorite electrolyte solution to a gallon of your filtered water. This helps to "re-mineralize" it.

Scrutinize your bottled waters, filters, purification systems and reverse osmosis systems, and choose a source for your most important fluid that you trust.

How much water?

Here are suggestions about water consumption for children. You can modify according to size, weight and energy or athletic requirements:

Daily Water Requirement	
Infants	8 to 20 oz.
School Age Children (ages 5-10)	20 to 50 oz.
Adolescents, Teens, Adults	48 to 80 oz.

Generally, the number of ounces of water a child or adult should consume per day is about one half his or her body weight. For example, if a child weights 60 pounds, his or her daily consumption of water should be 30 ounces, about one quart or one liter.

To learn more about bottled water, check www.fda.gov, as the FDA is the regulating agency for this type of water. For regulations about tap water, check www.epa.gov for the Environmental Protection Agency regulations.

---

1. *Adams PF, Hendershot GE, Marano MA. Current estimates from the National Health Interview Survey, 1996. National Center for Health Statistics. Vital Health Stat. 1999; 10(200).*

2. *"Cancer Statistics, 2007", Ahmedin Jemal, DVM, PhD; Rebecca Siegel, MPH; Elizabeth Ward, PhD; Taylor Murray; Jiaquan Xu; Michael J. Thun, MD, MS, CA Cancer J Clin 2007;57:43–66*
3. *"Factors Associated With Difficult Toilet Training", Alison Schonwald, MD, Lon Sherritt, MPH, Ann Stadtler, CPNP and Carolyn Bridgemohan, MD, Pediatrics, Vol. 113 No. 6 June 2004, pp. 1753-1757.*
4. *"Gut as the largest immunologic tissue", Takamura, S., M. Niikura, T.-C. Li, N. Takeda, S. Kusagawa, Y. Takebe, Journal of Parenteral and Enteral Nutrition, Sept/Oct 1999, 23:S7-S12.*
5. *Gershon, M.D. Michael: The Second Brain, Harper Collins, New York, NY 1998*
6. *"Prebiotics, Probiotics, and Symbiotics Affect Mineral Absorption, Bone Mineral Content, and Bone Structure", Katharina E. Scholz-Ahrens, Peter Ade, Berit Marten, Petra Weber, Wolfram Timm, Yahya Ail, Claus-C. Glüer and Jürgen Schrezenmeir, Journal of Nutrition 137:838S-846S, March 2007*
7. *Bland, PhD, Jeffrey: Solve Digestive Problems with Probiotics, New Hope Natural Media, Boulder, CO 1995*
8. *Gut as the largest immunologic tissue, Takamura, S., M. Niikura, T.-C. Li, N. Takeda, S. Kusagawa, Y. Takebe, Journal of Parenteral and Enteral Nutrition, Sept/Oct 1999, 23:S7-S12.*
9. *Batmanghelidj, F: The Body's Many Cries for Water, Global Health Solutions, Inc. Falls Church, VA 1995*
10. *To check what contaminants have been found in your local water system, log on to The National Tap Water Database at www.ewg.org/tapwater/.*
11. *"Storage time increases antimony in bottled water", Environmental Science & Technology Online, Science News, January 24, 2007*

PART TWO - THE CHALLENGES: Hidden Toxins and Beyond

Chapter Four

FOOD: Power-Less

IT SHOULD NOT HARM US

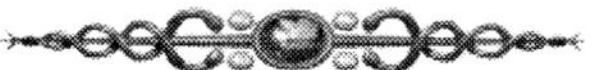

Simple and easy is the name of the game these days. With working parents the dilemma is: how do I prepare three healthy and solid meals a day for my family? Schedules are crazy, so we reach for something that is fast and stress-free. Frozen food in bags and boxes, packages on the shelf, cans and bottles are often our choices. And they come with long ingredient lists. Who has the time to read them? Who can pronounce them and what do they mean? Let's start with deciphering labels and knowing <u>what's</u> really in your food. Most of the details about the following toxins are suppressed; you have to dig deep to find validating studies. But here they are:

Preservatives/Additives

These prevent food from spoiling and are used to make it more 'appealing'. They are found in many cereals, crackers, cookies, processed meats and even chewing gum.

BHA - Butylated hydroxyanisole or BHA is a preservative and antioxidant added to foods to prevent fats from becoming rancid. It is phenol-based, from petroleum and has been found to cause allergic reactions in sensitive individuals.[1] BHA is associated with liver toxicity, promotion of tumors and exacerbation of behavioral problems.[2] It is found in butter, meat, cereals, chewing gum, potato chips, dehydrated potatoes and beer.

BHT – Butylated hydroxytoluene or BHT is also a phenol compound, derived from petroleum. It has antioxidant properties and is used to preserve fats, flavorings, colors, and odor. It is also added to cosmetics and body care products to preserve the oils. Some studies indicate a link between BHT and hyperactivity and behavior disturbances. Other studies show a link with cancer.[3] BHT is also added to shortening, cereals, potato chips and some packaging materials.

TBHQ – Tertiary butylhydroquinone or TBHQ is a phenol-based antioxidant, similar to BHA and BHT. It is typically used in frozen fish products, powdered dairy products, peanuts and cosmetics. As it is effective in stabilizing unsaturated fats and polyunsaturated frying oils, TBHQ is often used as a preservative for fast food French fries, to extend the use of the oil. It is also sprayed on chicken "nugget"- type foods. Some studies in animals indicate that TBHQ may cause cancer.[4] Like BHA and BHT, it is derived from petroleum and has been associated with learning and behavior problems.[5]

Phosphates are used in carbonated drinks, baking powder, cake mixes, donuts, cheese, canned meats, crab and tuna, hot dogs, puddings, dry cereals, French fries, chocolate milk and orange juice. Phosphates are used for color stabilization, leavening enhancement, decreasing cooking time and improving emulsification. They have been found to cause learning problems and oppositional behavior. Over-consumption may also result in calcium deficiencies.[6]

Nitrates and Nitrites are found in processed meat, preserved poultry, and especially pork. They may worsen symptoms of asthma, irritability, hyperactivity and insomnia. Nitrates and nitrites have been found to cause headaches.[7] They can also react with amino acids and produce nitrosamine which is a known carcinogen or cancer-causing agent.[8]

Sulfur and Sulfites – Sulfur dioxide is used as a preservative in dried fruits such as apricots and raisins. It is used as an anti-brown agent for French fries, fresh fruits, molasses, and in some marmalade. Treatment with sulfites can destroy essential nutrients, such as thiamine (vitamin B1). Problems related to sulfite consumption include stomach aches, hives and asthma. Sulfites or sulfur dioxide have been banned by the FDA for use on salad bars, because some people have died from anaphylactic shock due to their exposure. Some foods that still contain sulfites are deli meats, cake and cookie mixes, instant potatoes, lemon juice concentrates and alcoholic beverages, especially red wine. Common allergic reactions to sulfites are headaches, red ears, hot hands and hot feet.

Sodium Benzoate is a preservative that has been used for years to prevent microorganisms from growing in acid foods. It is only effective in highly acidic foods and beverages, so it is found in carbonated drinks, jams and preserves with citric acid, fruit juices, pickles and foods with vinegar such as salad dressings, soy sauce, Chinese mustard, and duck sauce. It will appear as "sodium benzoate" or "E211" on the label.[9] Sodium benzoate has recently been indicated as one of a mix of additives that can increase hyperactive behavior.[10]

It is important to realize that sodium preservatives can reduce the availability of potassium in the body. This can lead to electrolyte imbalance and dehydration, as well as hives, eczema, and asthma.

Flavorings: MSG and Vanillin

MSG is a neurotoxin responsible for "Chinese Restaurant Syndrome", causing heart palpitations, stomach aches, irritability, hyperactivity, chest pains numbness, cold sweats and restlessness. It is found in soups and hidden in products such as bouillon, gravies and sauces. It is often termed "natural flavors" or autolyzed yeast. If you see HVP on a label, it probably contains MSG. HVP or hydrolyzed vegetable protein is a flavor enhancer used in instant soups, frankfurters, sauce mixes and beef stews. Hydrolyzed soy protein contains MSG, as well. Think of it this way – if it has to be used, it is probably substituting for the real flavor lost in the processing.[11]

Taste substitutes aside, the more serious problems with MSG are toxicity to the brain and central nervous system. In his book, *Excitotoxins: The Taste That Kills*, Dr. Russell Blaylock discusses the repercussions of MSG on the body: seizures, neurological disorders, learning disabilities, headaches, hormone imbalances and allergies.[12]

Especially alarming, are results from a study at the University of Liverpool, where researchers found that when blue dye was combined with MSG, damage to nerve cells was 4 times greater than when the additive was tested alone.[13] Read labels cautiously because MSG is something to avoid.

Vanillin: Another harmful flavor enhancer is vanillin, formulated to imitate the taste of vanilla. Vanillin has been found to have many toxic effects. Studies indicate that it blocks a certain enzyme in the liver which breaks down neurotransmitters, such as dopamine, serotonin and noradrenaline. This may result in an abnormal build-up of these brain chemicals, tipping the emotional, behavioral and cognitive scales.[14]

In other words, a food that contains vanillin can actually prevent proper brain function. The repercussions, of course, are very far-reaching because the neurotransmitters control emotional states, behavior, sleep, energy, memory and so many other mental processes.

Vanillin is widely used in products labeled "vanilla", as well as chocolate. People who think they are allergic to chocolate may actually be reacting to the vanillin flavoring it contains, and not the chocolate itself. A good experiment would be to find a chocolate free of this additive and test your sensitivity to it.

Many flavorings contain vanillin as part of their formula. Check out the following list of ingredients of a synthetic raspberry flavoring: Vanillin, Ethylvanillin, Alphaionone, Maltol, 1-(p-hydroxyphenyl)-3-Butanone, Dimethyl Sulphide, 2,5-Dimethyl-N-(2-pyrazinyl) Pyrrole. Many of these chemicals are derived from petroleum. What's even more bizarre is ... where's the fruit?[15]

Colorings

Artificial colorings are found in most processed foods, over-the-counter and prescribed medications, and cosmetic and body-care products. They are chemical dyes labeled FD&C red, yellow and blue, followed by a number (FD&C red #40). The "D&C" indicates that the certified colors can be used only in drugs and cosmetics. Though they are labeled as GRAS (Generally Regarded As Safe), they are highly toxic and have been shown to be as such in many studies.[16] The FDA has certified a list of permissible amounts of contaminants such as mercury and lead allowed in products for children. The colors permitted in drugs and cosmetics may have twice the lead contaminant allowed in foods.[17] Derived from petroleum, artificial coloring can cause red ears, red cheeks, skin rashes, hyperactivity, irritability, decreased attention span, anger and aggression. Foods that contain colorings are cereals, fruit drinks, candy, cake decorations, hot dogs, bologna, margarine and some butter. Gee, you can even buy blue and green catsup today. Other products containing colorings are cough syrups, children's vitamins, many over-the-counter and prescription medications. Artificial colorings are highly prevalent in cosmetics, toothpaste and other body care products.

Artificial Sweeteners

Artificial sweeteners were originally developed so that manufacturers could sweeten food more economically. The hype is of course, that artificially sweetened foods and drinks contain fewer calories and don't cause a rise in blood sugar levels. Funny, that with all the consumption of these artificial sweeteners, diabetes is at an all-time high and as a society, we are fatter than ever. Something's not working. These chemicals are toxic and may potentially cause metabolic imbalances, counterproductive to our goals.

Aspartame, NutraSweet, Equal, Equal Measure, Spoonful, Canderal (E951) are all names for the same substance, aspartame. They contain neurotoxins, which can change the neurotransmitter output in the brain, specifically norepinephrine, epinephrine and dopamine. These changes can negatively impact emotions, behavior and cognitive function.[18]

They can damage nerve and brain cells. The FDA has received many complaints about aspartame (trade name is NutraSweet) in regards to headaches, memory loss, seizures, focus problems, liver toxicity and tumors, but has not banned the substance.[19,20]

It is important to realize that aspartame is contained in many over-the-counter and prescribed medications for children. Some examples are Pedialyte, Pedialyte frozen pops, Augmentin, the prescribed pediatric antibiotic, children's vitamins, other OTC products and prescription medications.

A new version of aspartame, called Neotame is also made by NutraSweet Co. and was approved by the FDA in 2002. It is 8,000 times sweeter than table sugar and 40 times sweeter than aspartame. It is supposedly more chemically stable and therefore more "bake-able".[21] The jury is still out on this, but no chemical is good to ingest, so I'm sure there will be negative information out on this in the future.

Splenda and Sucralose were developed from chlorinated sucrose. Though they haven't yet been adequately tested, no food that is chlorinated can possibly be good. Also, sucralose has been found to contain many other chemicals, such as toluene and formaldehyde.[22] Results of long-term use in humans has not been established.

Saccharin or Sweet 'n Low is derived from petroleum and toluene, two very toxic chemicals. One study has indicated that taken in high doses, it can lead to bladder cancer. It is not recommended for children.[23]

Sunette, Sweet and Safe, and Sweet One are different names for the same artificial sugar substitute, Acesulfame-k. It is found in chewing gum, dry mixes for beverages, instant coffee and tea, gelatin desserts, puddings, non-dairy creamers, sports drinks and athletic products. This substance is inadequately tested and preliminary research points to it being a potential carcinogen.

Pesticides, Chemical Fertilizers

Most of the vegetables and fruits today are grown in soil that has been fertilized with chemicals, sprayed with pesticides and herbicides, waxed with chemicals and sometimes injected with dyes. All these chemical substances are ingested when our kids eat salads, drink orange juice, have an apple after lunch, and so on.

It is more imperative than ever to --- Buy Organic! This will reduce the amount of chemical intake from your food. Most grocery stores and all health food stores now have organic produce sections. Many towns in North America offer farmers' markets where local farmers sell local, organically grown food. The following information will help you purchase the purest and least toxic food for your family.

Fruits and Vegetables: Most likely to be contaminated

Pesticides and herbicides are used to kill insects on growing plants, especially fruits and vegetables. But these chemicals can also change and kill living cells in both humans and animals, when ingested. When cells are changed or mutated, they can grow out of control and lead to conditions such as cancer of the liver, lung, pancreas, small and large intestines, or stomach. Pesticides also interfere with the manufacture of hormones and are toxic or poisonous to the brain and nervous system. While washing and rinsing fresh produce may reduce levels of some pesticides, it does not always eliminate them.

Buying organic produce is imperative in order to reduce health risks. It is almost impossible to wash off pesticides entirely from most foods. It is also difficult to ensure that foods imported from other countries are safe, as they often do not have laws controlling pesticide use. If buying organic is too expensive or the food is not readily available, try to obtain a good produce-washing product from your local health food store. Another good strategy is to avoid the top 20 pesticide-contaminated foods, and look for the least contaminated.

Below is a list of produce with the highest level of pesticide contamination from the Environmental Working Group, Washington. D.C.[24]

Top 20 foods, most likely to be highly contaminated with pesticides:

- Apples*
- Cauliflower
- Celery*
- Cherries
- Cucumber
- Grapefruit
- Grapes-Imported & Dom
- Green Beans
- Lettuce
- Mangoes
- Mushrooms-Button
- Nectarines*
- Oranges
- Papayas
- Peaches*
- Pears
- Peppers-Hot
- Peppers-Sweet Bell*
- Plums
- Potatoes
- Red Raspberries
- Spinach
- Strawberries*

***Peaches, nectarines, apples, strawberries, celery and bell peppers are the top six foods, most likely to be contaminated with pesticides.**

Waxes from paraffin are applied to fruit or vegetables to seal in the pesticides and fungicides used to kill insects and keep them from damaging the crops. Scrubbing may help; peeling is better. Organic and wax-free is best. The two most heavily waxed foods are cucumbers and tomatoes. Other waxed foods are apples, citrus fruits, eggplant, peppers, rutabagas, parsnips and turnips.

Almonds & Sunflower Seeds can hold more pesticides because they and other chemicals have an affinity for the lipids or fats in the nuts and seeds. Buy these fresh, raw and organic.

Some fruits such as **papayas and mangoes** have very thin skins and absorb pesticide sprays more deeply causing higher levels of chemical contamination. These are called systemic pesticides; you can't wash them away – they are pervasive and they toxify our bodies. Purchase the organic versions of these foods, whenever possible. Your local health food store will most likely carry organic cereals, breads, cookies and other grocery items. Many conventional grocery stores have natural food sections and these are expanding as their consumers become more health conscious.

Rice is the most frequently consumed food on the planet. Although the herbicide 2,4,5-T was banned in 1984, it and many persistent water-soluble insecticides have been found to contaminate the ground water near prominent rice fields, so we suggest purchasing organic rice.

Potential Problems with Other Foods

Pesticides are pervasive and stored in higher amounts in the fats of food; dairy products tend to retain higher levels of residues and chemicals from feeds.

Corn is heavily treated with the herbicide atrazine (a known hormone disrupter) and it is also sprayed after harvesting.

Eggs are one of the most bio-available proteins but are often contaminated with salmonella bacteria because of the unhygienic, crowded conditions of the farm. Factory farm chickens are also given antibiotics. The best option is organic, free range, free of antibiotics.

Leafy Greens - Lettuces, Spinach, Kale and Chard: Sprayed chemicals tend to remain on the leaves of these vegetables. In FDA studies, spinach was the most frequently found leafy green to contain the more potent pesticides, especially the organophosphates (neurotoxins) and permethrin (noted as mildly carcinogenic).

Milk is a common source of the herbicide atrazine (a known endocrine hormone disrupter) and the growth hormone BGH which has been genetically engineered to boost milk production in the animals.

Wheat is one of the most heavily treated grains because it is stockpiled as a basic commodity and fumigated periodically to keep down pests. It has been suggested that some forms of so-called wheat allergy, which have been associated with learning problems and difficulty in concentrating, may actually be a neurotoxin reaction to the pesticide residues in the grain.

Grains, including rice are often bleached to give them a clean, white color.

The following foods are not highly contaminated

- Asparagus
- Broccoli
- Brussels sprouts
- Cabbage
- Carrots
- Corn - frozen sweet
- Onions - green & yellow
- Pineapple
- Sweet peas - frozen
- Sweet potatoes
- Watermelons

The following foods are the least likely to be contaminated:

- Bananas
- Kiwi

Nutrients in Plants Affected by Pesticides

Organic plants have been shown to have higher mineral levels than non-organic plants.[25] Studies also indicate that vitamin levels of plants treated with certain pesticides are significantly lower. This is different than the notion that plants raised with chemicals are low in nutrients because the soil is depleted. Rather, the chemicals actually reduce the amount of nutrients in the plants after application.[26]

The nutrients most often affected are vitamin C, beta carotene and the B vitamins. The irony is that these vitamins are the very ones required by our defense systems in order to withstand the onslaught of chemical toxins. Vitamin C has been well documented in the prevention and treatment of cancers. Beta carotene has been shown to strengthen the immune system and protect from many degenerative illnesses. Also, be aware that toxins from pesticides can accumulate and lodge in the fat tissues and organs of our bodies. This is not something that we necessarily feel. We need to encourage their elimination – and avoid them to begin with.

In summary, try to purchase the organic versions of the fruits and vegetables that your family eats a lot. This is a way to keep the majority of your foods organic. It is more costly, but in the long run, the health savings outweighs the monetary output.

Caffeine

This stimulant is contained in colas, root beer, coffee, iced teas (black tea), chocolate, dessert or snack foods that contain chocolate and many energy drinks and sports drinks. It can cause hyperactivity, irregular heartbeat, anxiety, depression, mood swings, hypoglycemia, insomnia, malabsorption, acid reflux, diarrhea and fatigue.

"Caffeine - Exposed: Soda Labels Show the Good, the Bad and the Ugly"
Schan, S, ABC NEWS, March 29, 2007.
http://www.abcnews.go.com/Health/Diet/story?id=2990014&page=1

-- Caffeine is a nervous system stimulant and can speed up your metabolic rate, increase energy and open up air-way passages.
-- When caffeine is used excessively, the adrenal hormone system can be thrown off balance. Resulting symptoms may be nervousness, irritability, insomnia, dizziness, fatigue, headaches, heartburn, anxiety, hypertension and palpitations.

How Much Is Too Much? High intake of caffeine is 500 mg daily. Medium is between 250-500 mg and a low intake is below 250 mg. Here is a list of caffeine amounts:

- Coca Cola Classic -- 34.5mg (12-ounce can)
- Diet Pepsi -- 36mg (12-ounce can)
- Pepsi -- 37.5mg (12-ounce can)
- Diet Coke -- 46.5mg (12-ounce can)
- Mountain Dew -- 54mg (12-ounce can)
- Diet Pepsi Max -- 69mg (12-ounce can)
- Instant Coffee -- 40-105mg (150ml cup)
- Filtered Coffee -- 110-150mg (150ml cup)
- Tea -- 20-100mg (150ml cup)
- Starbucks Coffee, Grande -- 500mg (16-ounce cup)
- Chocolate Cake -- 20-30mg (one slice)

- Caffeine Pill -- 50-200mg (read label to determine exact dose)

The negative effects mentioned above can occur with as little as 100 mg caffeine intake daily. You might want to taper your intake.

Allergic Foods

A food to which a person has an allergic reaction is an allergic food for them. An allergic reaction can be anything from nasal congestion, throat congestion, ear congestion, watery eyes or nose, to a skin rash or even flu-like symptoms. This is an immune reaction. The common foods that children and adults are allergic to are sugar, dairy, wheat, gluten-containing grains, soy, corn, tomato, eggs, oranges, chocolate, shellfish, peanuts and tree nuts.

Sensitivities

Other foods may cause digestive or behavioral/emotional reactions, which are labeled 'sensitivities'. These may include any of the above allergens as well as chemical additives and pesticides. A common substance that causes reactions is called a salicylate. There is a complete program, called the Feingold Program, which outlines all the natural and chemical salicylates that can cause physical, behavioral and emotional reactions. Some of the natural foods are apples, oranges, almonds and berries. They may seem innocuous but do contain natural salicylates, which some people must avoid. Chemical salicylates include BHA, BHT, food colorings, flavorings like MSG and vanillin, and artificial sweeteners. Some people, especially children are hyper-sensitive to salicylates and they experience problems with behavior, focus and concentration. Others may not have obvious effects, but these chemicals are toxins and we would all do well to avoid them. (See *Feingold Diet Chapter 11*.)

"Bad Fats"

Bad fats are ingredients and foods such as heated oils, trans fats in margarine, cottonseed and partially hydrogenated oils, fried foods and fast foods such as burgers, French fries, chicken nuggets and fish sandwiches. These bad fats impair the absorption of the good fats needed for proper brain function, and they can lead to liver, gall bladder, cardiovascular and weight problems. (See *Chapter 2 on Fat Facts*.) Also, Olestra or Olean is a fat substitute that was developed to help prevent heart disease. It is used in chips and crackers, mostly, but is indigestible. The unfortunate response though, is one of flatulence and diarrhea. Also, this ingredient causes malabsorption of the fat soluble carotenoids like beta carotene, lutein and lycopene. Not a good bet – it backfires, literally!

Modern Cooking Methods

Boiling vegetables and frying foods such as potatoes and meats or seafood destroys the vitamins and the fatty acids that they contain. Thus the food becomes more "empty" or the nutrients are not absorbable, or both. When food is heated by fire, the molecules rub against each other causing friction. When microwaves heat food, the electromagnetic field is altered.

The magnetic polarity of the atoms is alternated: positive becomes negative and negative becomes positive.[27] This happens thousands of times per second. Studies have shown that microwaving protein foods changes the L-form amino acids into D-form amino acids that are not absorbable and lead to the production of free radicals that cause degenerative diseases.[28] Also, using plastic wrap and plastic containers forces plastic molecules into the food. Use only glass or ceramic containers.[29]

Phenolic Compound Contents in Edible Parts of Broccoli Inflorescences after Domestic Cooking

F Vallejo, F, Tomás-Barberán, FA, García-Viguera, C, Laboratorio de Fitoquimica, Dep. de Ciencia y Tecnología de los Alimentos, Murcia, Spain, 30 January 2003 (Society of Chemical Industry)

In this research article, a comparison of cooking methods of fresh, raw broccoli reveals the following loss of nutrients:

- Microwave: 97% of flavonoids lost
- Boiling: 66% of flavonoids lost
- Pressure cooking: 47% of flavonoids lost
- Steaming: minimal flavonoids lost

In conclusion, a greater quantity of bioflavonoid compounds is provided by consuming steamed broccoli as compared with broccoli prepared by other cooking processes.

It is obvious from this study that steaming vegetables is the best choice because it leaches the least amount of nutrients, compared to other forms of cooking.

Sugar

Sugar is a common culprit of behavior and emotional imbalances, causing moodiness, hyperactivity, depression, irritability, fatigue, and blood sugar irregularities. The incidence of childhood diabetes is at its highest today. This is largely due to over-consumption of soda, fruit drinks, milk, snack foods and desserts. They all contain sugar: high fructose corn syrup, fructose, lactose, white sugar and so many others.

From infancy, we develop a taste for sweet things because commercial infant formulas and baby foods even contain sugar. Additionally, sugar has a negative impact on certain white blood cells, the neutrophils, thereby weakening the immune system. Vulnerability to colds, flues, ear infections and respiratory illnesses may result. See C*hapter 9* for information about natural sweeteners -- better choices.

GMO's

GMO's are genetically modified organisms created by genetic engineering and are contained in a multitude of commercial foods on the market today. Genetic engineering is a technology used to create whole new life forms by splicing genes from one living organism with another.

Scientifically this may be exciting, but for the human body, the potential damaging effects are unlimited and unknown. In essence, crossbreeding between unrelated species takes place: between plants and animals, between bacteria and plants, and even between human genes and plants and animals.

The testing of these products is far too sketchy to take a chance on ingesting them in our every day diet. No long-term affects have been studied. GMO's can mutate and combine with other organisms, and potentially have far-reaching concerns for future generations. People with allergies may be the most susceptible. Common products that contain GMO's are: baby food, infant formulas, soybeans, cotton, potatoes, tomatoes, corn and pesticides. Most GMO foods are unlabeled.

Xenobiotics and Hormones

Xenobiotics and Hormones are man-made substances such as pesticides, industrial and automotive pollutants, as well as numerous household chemicals. We breathe them and we eat them every day. New studies indicate that these harmful chemicals contribute to degenerative illnesses and hormone imbalances.

Xenobiotics may also be called Xenoestrogens because they can cause hormone imbalances that affect the estrogen hormone levels in our bodies. They also enter our food supply through the use of antibiotics and hormones in animal products. This includes all animal flesh and dairy products that are not labeled organic or hormone-free.[30]

Food Additive Studies Show a Connection to Behavior & Learning Problems

Here is a list of scientific studies displaying the role that food additives and food allergies play in the brain function of our children – children with behavior and learning problems. These studies show a direct connection.

"Food additives and hyperactive behavior in 3-year-old and 8/9-year-old children in the community": a randomized, double-blinded, placebo-controlled trial.
McCann D, Barrett A, Cooper A, et al, *The Lancet,* 2007 Nov 3;370(9598):1560-7.

Fruit drinks with these additives were used:
Food colorings - sunset yellow, also known as E110; carmoisine, or E122; tartrazine, or E102; ponceau 4R, or E124; Preservative - sodium benzoate or E211
153 three-year-old and 144 eight- to nine-year-old children received a challenge drink containing sodium benzoate and 1 of 2 artificially colored mixes or a placebo mix. Special hyperactivity testing combined with teacher and parent ratings were used to assess the children's behavior.
"Artificial food colors and ... additives have long been suggested to affect behavior in children. These findings show that ... adverse effects of artificial colors and sodium benzoate were not just seen in children with extreme hyperactivity (such as ADHD), but ... also ... in the general population and across the range of severities of hyperactivity."

Positive Results on Behavior When Eliminating Food Coloring and Preservatives
Bateman, B. et al. "Artificial Food Coloring and Benzoate Preservative Challenge on Hyperactivity in a General Population of Preschool Children", *Archives of Disease in Childhood,* June 2004, 89: 506-511

Subjects: Four groups of 277 three-year-olds: 1) hyperactive, 2) allergic, 3) hyperactive and allergic, 4) normal.
Procedure:
1) Additive-free diet for 3 weeks.
2) Additive-laced (yellow #5 and benzoate) beverage vs. placebo daily
3) Double-blind; rated by parents
Results:
1) Hyperactivity decreased significantly with additive-free diet
2) All groups showed "increased behavior problems" on exposure days.

Foods and Additives are Common Causes of Attention Deficit/Hyperactive Disorder in Children Boris, M, Mandel, F, *Annals of Allergy*, May 1994, Vol. 72, pp. 462-8

"This study demonstrated a beneficial effect of eliminating reactive foods and artificial colors in diets of children with ADHD. Dietary factors may play a significant role in the etiology of the majority of children with ADHD."

The Impact of a Diet Low in Food Additives and Sugar on the Academic Performance in 803 New York City Public Schools
Schoenthaler, S, et al, *Internat'l Journal for Biosocial and Medical Research*, 1986, Vol.8(2), pp.18e475-195

"... lowered sugar (sucrose), synthetic food colors/flavors, and 2 preservatives (BHA & BHT) over 4 years in 803 public schools resulted in a 15.7% increase in the mean academic percentile rating..." **This study was done with one million students.**

Controlled Trial of Oligoantigenic Treatment in the Hyperkinetic Syndrome J. Egger et al, The Lancet, March 9, 1985

82% overactive children improved behaviorally. Headaches and abdominal pain also improved with a restricted diet eliminating artificial colors, preservatives, milk, eggs, chocolate, sugar, wheat, soy and oranges. (Double blind, placebo study)

Food Additives, Insomnia and Irritability
Rowe & Rowe, "Synthetic food coloring and behavior, a dose response effect in a double blind, placebo-controlled study", Journal of Pediatrics 1994; 125:691-8

Significant behavioral changes were noted when eliminating food dyes and additives. Irritability, restlessness and sleep disturbances occurred with re-introduction of a single dye, such as tartrazine.

Food Allergy Reactions In Hyperactive Children – results from two studies:

Item	Study #1 % Reacting	Study #2 % Reacting
Red dye	88	-
Yellow dye	80	-

Blue dye	80	-
Coloring and preservatives	-	79
Cow's milk	73	64
Soy	-	73
Chocolate	33	64
Grapes	40	50
Orange	40	45
Peanuts	47	32
Wheat	30	49
Corn	40	29
Tomato	47	20
Egg	20	40
Cane sugar	40	16
Apple	40	13
Fish	-	23
Oats	-	23

No result indicates that item was not tested. Egger, J, Carter, C., Graham, P., Gumley, D. and Soothill, J. "Controlled trial of oligoantigenic treatment in the hyperkinetic syndrome', Lancet, 1985, i. pp. 540-5. O'Shea, J and Porter, S., "Double-blind study of children with hyperkinetic syndrome treated with multi-allergen extract sublingually, J. Learn. Disabil. 1983 14, pp. 189-91.

"Synthetic Food Colorings and Hyperactivity"

Rowe, KS Au *Paediatric Journal*, April 1988, Vol. 24 (2), pp.143-7.

40 of 55 children (72%) put on a 6-week trial of the Feingold Diet (food additive elimination diet) "...demonstrated improved behavior." 26 of them (47.3%) remained improved following "liberalization" of the diet over a 3-6 month period. (double-blind)

Insomnia Improves With Elimination of Food Additives

Kaplan, B, et al, "Dietary Replacement in Preschool-Aged Hyperactive Boys", *Pediatrics*, 1989, Vol. 83, pp. 7-17.

Over half the subjects had reliable placebo effects when they ate a diet eliminating artificial colors, flavors, preservatives, MSG, chocolate and caffeine. The diet was also low in simple sugars. Halitosis, night awakenings and ability to fall asleep improved.

Food Dyes Affect Children's Performance on Tests
Swanson,J, Kinsbourne, M, "Food Dyes Impair Performance of Hyperactive Children on a Laboratory Learning Test", *Science Magazine*, March 28, 1980, Vol. 207, pp. 1485-7.

The performance of the hyperactive children on learning tests was impaired when they received the dye blend, relative to their performance after they received the placebo. The performance of the non-hyperactive group was not affected by the challenge..."

---

1. *www.feingold.org*
2. *"The effect of butylated hydroxyanisole and butylated hydroxytoluene on behavioral development of mice." Stokes JD, Scudder CL, Dev Psychobiol 1974 Jul;7(4):343-50.*
3. *"The mouse rasH2/BHT model as an in vivo rapid assay for lung carcinogens." Umemura T, Kodama Y, Hioki K, Nomura T, Nishikawa A, Hirose M, Kurokawa Y. Jpn, Journal Cancer Res. 2002 Aug;93(8):861-6.*
4. *(Gharavi N, El-Kadi A (2005). "tert-Butylhydroquinone is a novel aryl hydrocarbon receptor ligand". Drug Metab Dispos 33 (3): 365-72. PMID 15608132*
5. *"The effect of butylated hydroxyanisole and butylated hydroxytoluene on behavioral development of mice." Stokes JD, Scudder CL, Dev Psychobiol 1974 Jul; 7(4):343-50.*
6. *www.phosadd.com*
7. *"Intolerance to Dietary Chemicals May Underlie Recurrent Headaches", Cornwell N, et al, Royal North Shore Hospital, Sydney Australia.*
8. *CA Cancer J Clin 2002;52:92-119*
9. *http://www.cspinet.org/reports/chemcuisine.htm ; FDA 2006 "Data on Benzene in Soft Drinks and Other Beverages, "United States Food and Drug "Food additives and hyperactive behaviour in 3-year-old and 8/9-year-old children in the community": a randomized, double-blinded, placebo-controlled trial. McCann D, Barrett A, Cooper A, Crumpler D, Dalen L, Grimshaw K, Kitchin E, Lok K, Porteous L, Prince E, Sonuga-Barke E, Warner JO, Stevenson J, Lancet. 2007 Nov 3; 370(9598):1560-7.ug Administration. Accessed June 2nd at: http://www.cfsan.fda.gov/~dms/benzdata.html*
10. *"Food additives and hyperactive behaviour in 3-year-old and 8/9-year-old children in the community: a randomized, double-blinded, placebo-controlled trial," McCann D, et al, Lancet, September 6, 2007 on line.*
11. *http://www.cspinet.org/reports/chemcuisine.htm*
12. *Blaylock, Russell, Dr., Excitotoxins: The Taste That Kills, Health Press, Dec 1996*
13. *Synergistic Interactions Between Commonly Used Food Additives in a Developmental Neurotoxicity Test. Lau K, McLean WG, Williams DP, Howard CV., Toxicol Sci. 2006 Mar;90(1):178-87, 2005 Dec 13; [Epub ahead of print]*

14. *"Common Food Additives are Potent Inhibitors of Human Liver 17 Alpha-Ethinyloestradiol and Dopamine Sulphotransferases", KJ Bamforth et al., Biochem Pharmacol 1993 Nov 17; 46(10); pp.1713-20).*
15. *www.feingold.org*
16. *www.feingold.org*
17. *www.feingold.org/Bluebook/page-06-7-more.pdf*
18. *"Direct and indirect cellular effects of aspartame on the brain", Humphries, P, Pretorius, E, Naudé, H, European Journal of Clinical Nutrition (2008) 62, 451–462; doi:10.1038/sj.ejcn.1602866; published online 8 August 2007*
19. *Blaylock, Russell, Dr., Excitotoxins: The Taste That Kills, Health Press, Dec 1996*
20. *Thompson, Dr. Laura Nelle, A Holistic guide to the Endocrine System, SCICN Press, Los Angeles, 1990*
21. *http://www.cspinet.org/reports/chemcuisine.htm*
22. *Pure Facts, Newsletter of the Feingold Assoc., Feb 2007, p.4.*
23. *CA Cancer J Clin 2002;52:92-119*
24. *www.ewg.org (Environmental Working Group)*
25. *Smith, B. 1993. Organic foods vs. supermarket foods: element levels. Journal of Applied Nutrition 45:35-39.*
26. *"Are Organic Foods Really Healthier For You?" Crinnion, Walter J, N.D, Organic Gardening Almanac, 1995; Llewelyn Pub.*
27. *Colbin, Annemarie: Food and Healing, Ballantine Books, NY, NY 1986*
28. *Diamond, John W. MD, Cowden, W. Lee, MD, Goldberg, Burton, Cancer: A Def Guide, p.100, Future Medicine Publishing, Tiburon, CA, 1997)*
29. *Weil, M.D., Andrew: 8 Weeks to Optimum Health, Alfred A Knophf, New York, 1997*
30. *Rapp, Doris J, MD, "Is This Your Child's World", Bantam Books, 1996*

~ ~ ~

Chapter Five

TOXIC METALS: How to Avoid Them, How to Eliminate Them

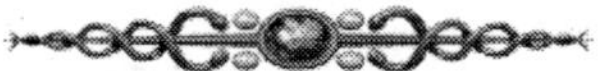

Heavy metal toxicity is a global problem. It is recognized as such, although low level, by government agencies including the Centers for Disease Control (CDC), Environmental Protection Agency (EPA), Food and Drug Administration (FDA) and many state health departments. It is astounding to me that we are rarely screened for this. That is why many alternative doctors advocate the use of toxic metal testing and programs for metal elimination.

We discuss here, types of testing for toxic metals and protocols for chelating and eliminating them. Treatment standards are needed but do not exist. Moreover, education about preventative measures for avoiding exposure is imperative. Groups most at risk for toxic metal exposure are:

- Those with occupational risks such as working with metals, paint, building materials, automobiles
- Pregnant mothers (should avoid metal exposure, i.e. dental work, seafood)
- Children (susceptible to metal exposure in utero and after birth and to metals from vaccinations)
- People exposed to dental materials
- Those with environmental exposure through contaminated water, soil, air
- Those who are aging (life-accumulation of metals in bone, kidneys, brain)

Which Metals?

There are several toxic and heavy metals that are relevant to autism and attention deficit disorders. The basic physical and mental health of all children and adults is at risk as well. The metals in question are: lead, mercury, aluminum, cadmium, arsenic and nickel.

Types of toxic effects in the body from metals:

- Neurotoxicity - damage to brain structures and brain chemicals
- Nephrotoxicity – damage to the kidneys, which filter and cleanse the blood
- Immune imbalances – hyper or hypo immune reactions (allergies, infections)

- Heart and cardiovascular – damage to the heart and circulatory vessels
- Bone and tissue deposits – build-up can cause arthritis and other structural problems
- Intestinal dysbiosis – overgrowth of bad bacteria, yeast or fungal myco-toxins
- Endocrine hormone disruption - thyroid, adrenal, sex hormones
- Cognitive problems – ADD, ADHD, depression, Alzheimer's, dementia
- Metabolic imbalances – fatigue and slowed metabolism, resultant weight gain

Lead – Lead is a proven neurotoxin. It has been linked to problems with learning and language development, leading to attention deficits, low vocabulary and poor reading skills. Lowered IQ, causing decreased school performance is also a potential result. High lead levels in the body can cause behavioral disorders such as aggression and oppositional defiance.

Lead toxicity in children can delay growth, impair motor skill development and cause poor hand-eye coordination. When lead lodges in the brain, it can affect the functions of the brain chemicals: dopamine, serotonin, and GABA. Cognitive, behavioral or emotional problems can result.

Pregnant women and young children are particularly vulnerable to lead exposure because lead easily crosses the placenta and may enter the fetal brain where it interferes with normal development. Lead has also been linked to miscarriage, reduced fertility in both, men and women, hormonal changes, menstrual irregularities and delays in the onset of puberty.

Nowadays, lead is usually absorbed into the body by drinking contaminated water or breathing polluted air. Water from lead pipes may be contaminated with lead. Fumes from lead-based paints, automobile exhaust, and polluted air from industrial plants or cigarette smoke may all contain lead.

Some cosmetics even contain small amounts. Lead-containing lipsticks, for instance, have recently been under scrutiny in the media. Over half of the brand-name lipsticks tested was found to exceed the .1 ppm limit (for candy). Most of these lipsticks were red. One application, of course, is not the problem. But applied several times per day and licked off the lips, lead-containing lipstick can cause cumulative toxicity.

> **"Lead poisoning associated with imported candy and powdered food coloring"**
>
> California and Michigan, *MMWR Morb Mortal Wkly Rep.* 1998 Dec 11; 47(48):1041-3.

> "Although the most common source of pediatric lead poisoning is dust within the home that contains deteriorated lead-based paint from walls and windowsills, other less common sources can result in excess exposure among children . . . This report describes two cases of pediatric lead poisoning associated with eating imported candy and food stuffs and underscores the importance of thorough history-taking to identify unusual sources of lead exposure."

The prevalence of lead in products manufactured in China has become very troublesome. From pencil pouches and metal craft jewelry to toy cars and video games, parents have yet one more area to be watchful about. Every month we hear about another toy or game that has been recalled due to lead levels, exceeding the safe limit.

Physical symptoms of elevated lead in both children and adults can manifest as abdominal pain, irritability, constipation and lack of hunger. In more progressive lead poisoning, a person may experience bone pain, gout, arthritis, anemia, memory loss and numbness or tingling in the extremities. New research also reveals that high lead levels are implicated in hypertension and high blood pressure.[1]

It is important to know that lead builds up in the body over time, so accumulation from multiple sources may go unnoticed. You wouldn't necessarily feel the effects of the contamination until later in life.

Mercury - Mercury is a toxic heavy metal, often found in the tissues of people with dental amalgams. Other contributors of mercury are contaminated fish, such as tuna, as well as latex wall paint, polluted water and certain vaccinations. Mercury toxicity may cause decreased attention span, irritability and anxiety. Learning disorders may result. Memory loss and fatigue are symptoms often reported by those with mercury toxicity.

This metal can also cross the placenta of a pregnant woman and the fetus may emerge contaminated. For this reason, pregnant women are advised to refrain from having dental work done. Certainly, it is important to avoid getting cavities filled or mercury amalgams removed during this time.

Mercury has been found in the cerebrospinal fluid of multiple sclerosis (MS) patients, at levels eight times higher than in the neurologically healthy controls, according to one scientific study. When the mercury is detoxified from the body, many people regain their muscle control and strength.[2,3,4]

Methyl Mercury - Coal-burning power plants are the largest human-caused source of mercury emissions to the air in the United States.[5] Burning hazardous wastes, producing chlorine, breaking mercury products, and spilling mercury, as well as the improper treatment and disposal of products or wastes containing mercury, can also release it into the environment.

Mercury in the air eventually settles into water or onto land where it can be washed into water. Once deposited, certain microorganisms can change it into methyl mercury, a highly toxic form that builds up in fish, shellfish and animals that eat fish. Fish and shellfish are the main sources of this volatile form of mercury exposure to humans. Methyl mercury builds up more in some types of fish and shellfish than others. The levels of methyl mercury in fish and shellfish depend on what they eat, how long they live and how high they are in the food chain.[6]

Seafood and Methyl Mercury

Fish and other seafood can play an important role in a good diet. Because fish are high in protein but low in unhealthy fats, they make a great alternative to red meat. Fish are also a good source of vitamins and minerals. Omega-3 oils are inherent in fish and are excellent for supporting brain function, immune and cardiovascular function.

The problem is that mercury, along with other metals, accumulates in the fatty tissue of fish and other seafood. So, some fish are healthier from this standpoint than others. Mercury does occur naturally in the environment. However, industrial pollution that reaches our lakes, streams, rivers and oceans ends up in the fish. The two worst pollutants, **mercury** and **PCB's**, have been linked to learning and memory problems in children, heart problems and possibly cancer.

Although some kinds of seafood contain too much mercury, others do not. By varying the kinds of fish in your diet and following certain portion guidelines, you can help protect your health and enjoy all the benefits of fish.

Canned tuna is the worst culprit, contributing to high mercury levels in children. Therefore, limiting portions is vital. Less than one ounce per twelve pounds of body weight per week is a good measure of tuna consumption for children. So, if a child is 36 pounds, then he or she should consume less than three ounces of canned tuna per week.

Avoiding albacore or white tuna is important across the board, as mercury levels are very high in these forms.[7]

Highest Level of Mercury

Big-eye Ahi	Orange Roughy	
King Mackerel	Shark	Tilefish
Marlin	Swordfish	

Moderately-High Levels of Mercury

Bluefish	Grouper	Spanish Mackerel
Canned Albacore Tuna	Sea Bass-Chilean	Yellow Fin Tuna
	Skate	

Moderate Levels of Mercury

Canned Light Chunk Tuna	Halibut	Sablefish
Carp	Lobster	Sea Trout
Cod-Alaskan	Mahi Mahi	Snapper
Croaker	Monkfish	Striped Bass
	Perch-Freshwater	

Lowest Levels of Mercury

Anchovies	Flounder	Sardines
Calamari	Freshwater Trout	Scallops
Canned Light Tuna	Herring	Shrimp
Catfish	Pollock	Tilapia
Domestic Crab	Salmon (wild)*	Whitefish

Note: *Not wild, but farmed salmon may contain PCB's, chemicals with serious long-term health effects.

In February 2004, the EPA revealed that about 630,000 children are born each year at risk for lowered intelligence and learning problems caused by exposure to high levels of mercury in the womb. Therefore, the FDA and the EPA are advising women who may become pregnant, pregnant women, nursing mothers and young children to avoid some types of fish and eat fish or shellfish that are lower in mercury.[8]

Dentistry and the Use of Mercury

Probably the most controversial issue concerning mercury toxicity is in the world of dentistry. Most dental amalgams or fillings contain mercury and are poisonous. About 98 percent of the North American population develops cavities, and mercury amalgams are packed into four fifths of them. Common symptoms of mercury poisoning are arthritis and inflammation, cardiovascular disease, digestive problems, dementia and allergies. Psychosomatic, unknown or mysterious conditions often related to allergies may clear up after the mercury amalgams are removed from the mouth.

Mercury Vapor - Vapor from mercury is very toxic and can be released from your dental amalgams or silver fillings as they corrode over time. These amalgams are typically a combination of mercury, sliver, copper, zinc, tin and other trace metals.

Mercury vapor is 100 percent absorbed at low dose and 74 percent absorbed at higher levels. It accumulates in critical organs: brain, kidneys, and also transfers across the placental membrane into the fetus. Where does it come from?

Common oral habits greatly increase the amount of mercury released and absorbed:

- Chewing gum
- Clenching teeth
- Grinding teeth[9]

Although mainstream dentistry does not agree that the mercury amalgams are causing so many problems, there are some dentists who believe the best thing to do is to remove the amalgams. This must be done very precisely by someone who knows and understands the process because mercury can slip into the body when the amalgams are being removed. Most dentists who do this procedure are called biological or mercury-free dentists and they often test replacement substances for their compatibility in your mouth.[10]

The world of biological dentistry opens many options in this realm. To find a biological dentist in your area, see the website: www.iaomt.org.

Cadmium - Cadmium is also a very toxic metal. Symptoms of cadmium toxicity are sore joints, decreased appetite, slow growth, zinc deficiency and kidney stones. The highest contributor to cadmium toxicity is cigarette smoke. It is found in cured tobacco and is toxic for both the smoker and the non-smoker. First hand and second hand smoke are high sources of cadmium.

Other cadmium sources are well water, some soft water, evaporated milk and some organ meats such as kidney and liver. Water from cadmium pipes can be a source, as well as fungicides sprayed on apples, tobacco, and potatoes. Cadmium can weaken the immune system and allow bacteria, viruses, yeast and parasites to proliferate.

In summary, toxic levels of cadmium may occur from:

- Breathing contaminated air from battery manufacturing, metal soldering or welding
- Eating contaminated shellfish, liver, kidney meats
- Breathing cigarette smoke
- Drinking contaminated water

Aluminum - Today, aluminum is everywhere ....under your arms, in your teeth and on your baby's skin. Anti-perspirants, toothpaste, dental amalgams, baby powder, cosmetics and cigarette filters contain aluminum.

We ingest it in drinking waters, commercial teas, cheeses, white flour, baking powder, aspirin and table salt. We cook with it, too; some pots and pans contain aluminum. Unfortunately, many over-the-counter and prescription antacids for digestive problems contain aluminum, as well.

Aluminum may also leach out of aluminum foil or cans into food and beverages. Sodas (with phosphoric acid), tomato sauce, pineapple and coffee in aluminum cans are major culprits, as well as food wrapped in aluminum foil. Commercial tomato sauces are often prepared in huge aluminum pots and the acidity of the tomatoes may cause leaching of aluminum from the cookware into the finished product. Coffee prepared in aluminum pots and pans may be very toxic.

Heavy coffee drinkers may also be at risk another way. It is speculated that because coffee drinking causes an acidic reaction in the digestive tract, aluminum contained in any food or drug may become toxic or more toxic because the acid will cause it to collect in the bloodstream. There, it can be carried to the brain along with the very blood that's supposed to nourish the brain cells. Aluminum has been implicated for years in several brain and neurological diseases, such as Alzheimer's and multiple sclerosis.[11]

It is sometimes found excreted in the stool, urine and hair of children diagnosed with ADHD, ADD and those with seizures. Hyperactivity, memory disturbances and learning disabilities may result from even mildly elevated levels of aluminum. Inhibition of neurotransmission and impaired motor coordination may also result. Senior citizens with extreme memory loss, absent-mindedness or dementia should be tested for aluminum levels. Science has been linking elevation of aluminum in the body with Alzheimer's disease for years. Studies have shown that the more antiperspirant used, the higher the risk for developing Alzheimer's. The same held true for antacids.[12]

According to several reports in the *Journal of Pediatrics, the British medical journal*, and *the Lancet*, many infant formulas contain aluminum. It was revealed that human breast milk contained 5-20 micrograms per liter of aluminum, cow's milk-based formulas contained 20 times as much and soy-based formulas contained 100 times as much. So, human breast milk had the lowest concentrations, proving to be the safest.[13,14]

Physical symptoms of aluminum toxicity may be brittle bones or osteoporosis, as aluminum is stored in the bones. Kidney malfunction may also result, as the kidneys filter aluminum.

If you were to look in the *PDR* or *Physician's Desk Reference*, you would be appalled to see that many pharmaceutical drugs contain some form of aluminum. Just look at the ingredient lists. These drugs, contaminated with aluminum, are prescribed for our children and our grandchildren every day.

Arsenic: Our Soil, Our Water, Our Chickens? - Eyebrows rise when we talk about arsenic poisoning. No, someone hasn't slipped it into your tea. Well – not really, unless you make your tea with fluoridated tap water. Consider that 90 percent of the fluoride used to fluoridate U.S. water systems comes directly from the pollution-scrubbing systems of the phosphate fertilizer industry. Hydrofluorosilicic acid is the name of this bi-product and it contains arsenic, lead and mercury. So, we have topical exposure of arsenic through bathing and, of course, we ingest it if we drink tap water. In a letter to Congress on July 7, 2000, the National Sanitation Foundation International (NSFI) reported that arsenic occurred about five times more frequently than any other contaminant, according to its testing.[15]

The poultry industry also promotes a source of arsenic. It is found in Roxarsone, the most common arsenic-based additive used in chicken feed to promote growth, kill parasites and improve the color of chicken meat. It is normally benign, but under certain conditions that can occur within live chickens or on farm land, Roxarsone can convert to more toxic forms of inorganic arsenic. Several food suppliers have stopped using Roxarsone, including Tyson Foods, which is the largest poultry producer in the United States. Even so, 70 percent of the nine billion broiler chickens produced annually in the United States are fed this harmful additive.

Other food containing arsenic may come from arsenic-rich soils. Europe recently banned food grown in such soil. The U.S. has not. Arsenic can be found in food dyes as well. As far as seafood is concerned, mussels, oysters and some shrimp from coastal water may contain arsenic.

Arsenic is often inhaled through these sources:

- downwind of a power plant
- after the burning of arsenate-treated lumber and building materials
- old deck painting
- coal combustion
- insect sprays and pesticides

Now for the toxic effects of arsenic. It has been linked to prostate, bladder, lung, skin, kidney and colon cancers. Low-level exposure can cause partial paralysis and diabetes. Other potential symptoms of arsenic toxicity are abdominal pain, gas, cramping, vomiting, chronic anemia, consistent low red or white blood cell count, garlicky odor to the breath, hyper-pigmentation of nails and skin, muscle aches, spasms and weakness.

Nickel - Nickel toxicity has been associated with industrial pollution, automotive pollution, cadmium-nickel batteries, fertilizers, cigarette and cigar smoke, metal jewelry and stainless steel utensils. Also, nickel is frequently used as a catalyst in the hydrogenation process; therefore, margarine, vegetable shortening and other hydrogenated fats may contain nickel. Imitation whipped cream is one such food. Other foods that may contain nickel are tea, cocoa and coffee.

Physical symptoms of nickel toxicity may include dermatitis, rashes and eczema, as well as nasal canal and lung problems.

Total Load - What is totally unknown - is what can occur from the cumulative effects of metal load and the multiple metals in the body. What if a child has multiple exposures of, for example, mercury and lead? There are no studies being done on this very issue. But, you can imagine what the exponential negative effects could be.

Types of Toxic Metal Testing

Standardized testing for metals through the blood may not reveal any high metal levels. Problems may go unnoticed, unless more sensitive testing is run. The mediums used to perform this sensitive testing are hair, urine and stool. You'll be surprised at what is revealed with these forms of testing.

Hair Analysis - Some doctors like to run hair analyses for the kids, teens and adults who have been diagnosed with ADD, ADHD, autism and learning disabilities because it is a very simple collection process. Hair is an ideal tissue for sampling and testing. First, it can be cut easily and painlessly, and can be sent to the lab without special handling requirements. Second, clinical results have shown that a properly obtained sample can give an indication of mineral status and toxic metal accumulation following long term or even brief exposure. One problem with hair analysis is that of false negatives. Toxic metals may be present in the body, but not being excreted. Since the hair test measures those metals or minerals excreted, the test may not show what is being stored.

Urine Test for Heavy Metals – Challenged or Provoked - A 24-hour urine collection to measure which toxic metals are excreted is a highly effective test. If you do the "challenge", you ingest certain chelator substances, such as

DMSA, prior to your urine collection. The idea is-the challenge or chelating products encourage release of the metals into the urine being collected. (www.metametrix.com)

Fecal Metals Test - Stool testing for heavy metals is very simple because the specimen is collected in a single step. Analysis of elements in feces is important because for many toxic metals, fecal (biliary) excretion is the primary natural route of elimination from the body. Fecal analysis also provides a direct indication of dietary exposure to toxic metals.
(www.doctorsdata.com)

Types of Chelation

Now for the good news! Heavy and toxic metals can be detoxified. The body can eliminate these harmful toxins, although sometimes stubborn, with the use of various techniques. These techniques fall into several categories: I.V. chelation therapy, oral chelation, rectal chelation and chelation through the skin. In the first three types, a particular substance chelates, wraps around or "claws" the toxic metal in order to usher it out of the cells.

1. Intravenous or I.V. Chelation

I.V. Chelation therapy is the most sophisticated and expensive form of cellular detoxification. In one form of this chelation, a protein-like material called **EDTA** or ethylene diamine tetra acetic acid is injected slowly into the area and binds with or chelates the toxic and heavy metals. The body excretes them through the urinary tract or the bowel, so it encourages flow of toxins out of the cells, into the bloodstream and out of the body.

ACAM, the American College of Advancement in Medicine has compiled 3,539 laboratory and clinical journal articles about EDTA and chelation therapy. Although not generally accepted by the medical mainstream, chelation therapy has been very effective for heavy metal detoxification and calcification that causes vascular diseases, such as arteriosclerosis and Alzheimer's. It is highly accepted in many other countries. EDTA has a great affinity for lead and, therefore, is a known effective lead detoxifier. It is, however, not known to be a good mercury chelator.

DMPS (2,3-dimercapto-1-propanesulfonic acid sodium), also known as Dimovol, is a synthetic amino acid chelating agent of toxic and heavy metals, delivered intravenously. It is believed by many to encourage metal removal through the kidneys, liver and gastrointestinal tract.

2. Oral Chelation

Oral chelation therapy is simple to perform, as the chelating agent is taken by mouth. Oral chelators are found in powder, capsule, liquid or homeopathic form. A wide variety of products may be used effectively for oral chelation and are readily available from your health food store, your health care provider or from the manufacturer direct:

Blue-green algae, especially from the freshwater of Klamath Lake in Oregon, is an effective chelator. It contains uniquely high levels of chlorophyll and amino acids.
Bowel cleansers, psyllium powder, apple pectin, bentonite clay and prune powder help bind to metals.
Chlorella or green algae has been researched for years, especially in Japan for its ability to chelate toxic metals.
Cilantro, the herb and food (or spice often referred to as coriander), is excellent to use for the chelation process and detoxifying metals from the body. It is especially good for mercury detox.
DMSA or succinic acid is a sulfhydryl-containing compound taken orally in capsule form. It is commonly used to bind to lead, mercury and other metals within the cells.
EDTA or ethylene diamine tetra acetic acid can also be taken orally, in capsule form. It is known for binding metals on the cell's surface and in the blood, so it can be used effectively with DMSA.
Garlic removes harmful chemicals from the body.
Glutathione, especially in a liposomal base, oral or topical, is vital to enhance detoxification of metals from the body. Studies indicate that metal accumulation can persist when glutathione antioxidant levels are low.[16]
Kelp, a form of seaweed, removes toxic metals.
N-acetylcysteine enhances synthesis of glutathione for enhanced metal elimination.
NDF or Nano-colloidal Detox Factors is a combination of cilantro, enzymes – in a base of multiple strains of probiotics. It is a liquid, and is easily administered to children.

3. Rectal Chelation

Recent studies have indicated that rectal chelation is extremely effective, in fact, more effective and less expensive than I.V. chelation. A special rectal suppository called Detoxamin is easily inserted by the individual. Some parents show the child how to insert it or they insert it for them.

Each suppository delivers 750 mg Ca-EDTA. Rectal chelation is very effective with excellent absorption. It is considered to be safer than I.V. chelations because it is "lower dose", in that, use of three Detoxamin suppositories is equal to one I.V. EDTA chelation. This is very significant. Detoxamin has broad specificity metal-chelation abilities. Studies have shown that after a thirty-day administration, significant amounts of lead, arsenic, mercury, aluminum, cadmium and nickel are excreted through the feces and the urine.

(For more information, contact 1-877-656-4553 or www.Detoxamin.com.)

4. Other Forms of Chelation – Through the Skin

The feet – yes, the feet are another avenue for toxic metal excretion. This can be a simple form of adjunct chelation to accompany your chosen chelation program. Detox foot pads with highly absorptive extracts and binders are put on the bottom of the heels or feet, overnight. Kids will enjoy seeing the colors of the pads in the morning. Also, detox foot baths can be very effective and very soothing. They work on the principle of eliminating toxins by creating negative ions which draw positively-charged toxins out of the feet.

Infrared sauna treatments can be helpful as adjunctive therapy to forms of chelation, as the penetrating heat helps the body eliminate metals from the fat tissue.

Chelation is One Thing; Detoxification is Another

Although chelation is a vital step in eliminating metals from the body, care must be taken in order for those toxins to actually LEAVE. In other words, the eliminative systems of the body need to be supported and the kidney and bowel channels must be open, before you embark on a chelation program. This is why it is extremely important to work with a health care professional who understands chelation and the body's detoxification processes. Metals and other toxins can re-circulate in the body if they are chelated and not eliminated. This can cause a variety of toxic symptoms, discomfort and an unsuccessful chelation program.

Gentle massage and lymphatic drainage techniques are very helpful (and enjoyable) during a detoxification program. The lymph system is a network of vessels with lymphatic fluid that carry the waste and toxics away from the cells to be eliminated. Jumping on a mini-trampoline is excellent for moving along the lymphatic fluid in the body and most kids like this part of the program best.

We must take these steps prior to chelation: Ensure hydration for cellular and kidney support. Ensure proper electrolyte or mineral balance, in order to improve cellular respiration. Make sure the bowels are moving fully, daily. Utilize antioxidants to avoid oxidative stress and prepare the body's ability to manufacture glutathione. This leads the way to proper detoxification and liver support. Enhance nutrient intake – vitamins, minerals, fatty acids. Work with a health practitioner who has expertise in this area. In conclusion, **read your labels** and scrutinize closely what goes into your mouths. Investigate your household products, get your well water tested and avoid the known sources of these toxic metals. If you or your health practitioner suspect there may be toxic metal accumulation, then, get a stool, urine or hair analysis test for confirmation. This will help determine the best course of treatment.

---

1. *Vaziri ND, Sica DA. Lead-induced hypertension; role of oxidative stress. Curr Hypertens Rep 2004; 6:314-320.*
2. *R.L. Siblerud et al,"Evidence that mercury from silver fillings may be an etiological factor in multiple sclerosis",Sci Total Environ,v142,n3, p191- 1994;*
3. *"Mental health, amalgam fillings, and MS", Psychol Rep,70(3 Pt2), 1992, 1139-51;*
4. *T.Engalls, Am J Forensic Med Pathol, 4(1):1983, Mar, 55-61.*
5. *http://epa.gov/mercury/about.htm.*
6. *www.nrdc.org - Natural Resources Defense Council*
7. *www.cfsan.fda.gov EPA-823-R-04-004 (Mar 2004)*
8. *WHO Environmental Health Criteria 118 (1991), section 5.1. General population exposure, Table 2, http://www.inchem.org/documents/ehc/ehc/ehc118.htm*
9. *Zamm AV. Removal of Dental Mercury: Often an Effective Treatment for the Very Sensitive Patient. J Orthomol. Med. 5(3):138-142, 1990.*
10. *"Brain Aluminum Distribution in Alzheimer's Disease and Experimental Neurofibrillary Degeneration", D. R. Crapper, S. S. Krishnan, A. J. Dalton, Science, 4 May 1973:Vol. 180. no. 4085, pp. 511 – 513.*
11. *American Journal of Epidemiology 2000;152:59-66*
12. *Aluminum content of milk formulae and intravenous fluids used for infants, McGraw, M, et al, Lancet, 1:157, 1986.*
13. *Aluminum Toxicity in Infants and Children: Pediatrics, Vol 78, 1986 1150-1154.*
14. *www.mercola.com*
15. *Arsenic in Chicken Production: Hileman, Bette, Chemical Engineering News, April 9, 2007, Vol 85, Number 15, pp 34-35.*
16. *Ahamed M, Verma S, Kumar A, Siddiqui MK. Environmental exposure to lead and its correlation with biochemical indices in children. Sci Total Environ 2005; 346:48-55.*

~ ~ ~

Chapter Six

VACCINATIONS: What You Need to Know

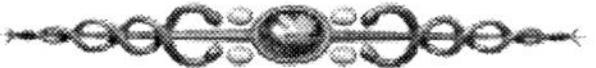

The following is information that can help you make the decision ...

To Vaccinate or Not to Vaccinate

Parents are often torn: "Should I have my child vaccinated or not?" "What other options do we have?" "Are there damaging agents in the vaccine preparations?" These are questions that many parents ask.

There is a great push to vaccinate our children. In spite of the fact that certain vaccinations may damage a child's brain, immune and nervous systems, most doctors, professionals and school officials urge parents to have their children vaccinated. They believe they are protecting the children. Most of them, however, have not been informed about the damage the vaccines can cause. These are the authorities that most parents believe.

If a parent questions vaccinating their child, what recourse do they have? Regulations about vaccinations vary from State to State and school to school.[1] At this time in the U.S., the laws on this topic are becoming more stringent. Sometimes it's a "do it, or else" situation! Either you have the child vaccinated or he or she can not attend the school. Parents and children may run the risk of being ostracized if they aren't vaccinated. Some parents are afraid to have their child play with a child who has <u>not</u> been vaccinated. The fear is pervasive; the fear is unwarranted.

So, parents are urged to vaccinate their children. They are fearful not to have them vaccinated, and yet there is mounting evidence that vaccinations may pose a great health risk to all children. This issue is not being sufficiently addressed in the mainstream medical community. We intend to expose in this chapter, information about toxic vaccine ingredients and specific health conditions that may result from vaccines. We will also discuss options for alternatives.

It is so important to be prepared for this event in your child's life. Vaccinating your children, or not vaccinating, is a personal decision, but it should be an informed one. To be armed with accurate information and know that you have options -- is to be fearless.

Vaccines vs. Immunity

A vaccination is used to create artificial immunity from a disease. It is the introduction of an antigen or toxoid on the skin, mucosal tissue or through injection, with the purpose of protecting the recipient from infection by a disease-causing agent. Immunization is the intended result from an injected vaccine. It is the process of inducing artificial immunity by administering an immuno-biologic agent. This agent is a preparation of killed microorganisms, living attenuated organisms or living fully virulent organisms administered to produce or artificially increase immunity to a particular disease. These are examples of artificial immunity.[2]

Natural immunity is just what it says – natural – and is more strengthening for the body than vaccines. It is the real thing. It is achieved when the body strengthens its immune system as it comes in contact with various pathogens. Immunity from disease often follows a single natural infection, whereas immunity from vaccines usually occurs only after several doses. There is no firm evidence that the administration of an immuno-biological agent or vaccine can bring about the development of adequate long-lasting immunity. Being vaccinated and having a strong immune system are two separate and distinct things.

The Problems with Vaccines ... They Contain Toxins

Along with immunobiologic agents or active ingredients, vaccines contain a wide variety of toxic and often harmful agents. Each vaccine has its own story – its own set of ingredients. For instance, despite what you may have heard, some flu shots still contain mercury in the form of the preservative, Thimerosal. For a chart of vaccines and their excipients and ingredients, see the website – www.ourchildrenshealth.com.

Toxic and heavy metals are found in many vaccines: mercury, lead, cadmium, antimony and aluminum. It is quite concerning that some children receive multiple vaccines in one visit and that may surpass the precautionary limit of that toxin, as determined by the Environmental Protection Agency (EPA).[3]

Commonly-Used Toxins That Occur in Vaccinations

Mercury - a toxic metal in the form of Thimerosal that causes cell death. It is contained in the Hepatitis B and DPT (Diphtheria, Pertussis or whooping cough, Tetanus) vaccines which are given at infancy and throughout childhood. Thimerosal is also a salicylate which is an aspirin-like compound, found to create toxic and allergic reactions in some children. It is present in some influenza vaccines. Mercury received by injection is more harmful than mercury received by ingestion.

Aluminum – found in vaccine adjuvants, which are components of vaccines designed to strengthen immunity or enhance antigen-specific responses.[4] Common adjuvants contain either aluminum hydroxide, aluminum phosphate or potassium aluminum sulfates and are found in the DTP, Hepatitis A and B, Polio, Anthrax, HPV and rabies vaccines. Aluminum is a metal, toxic to the brain and nervous system. It can cause seizures and memory loss.

Phenol - used as a disinfectant and dye with the potential of causing toxic or allergic reactions, found in Pneumovax, Hepatitis A and B.

Polysorbate 80 – a potentially toxic preservative found in DTaP, DTaP/HIB, HPV (Gardasil), Encephalitis vaccines.

Formaldehyde - a known cancer-causing agent and brain toxin present in many vaccines such as Hepatitis B, DPT, Polio and Anthrax.

Mycoplasma toxins have been found in certain vaccines. These have been implied as causes of several illnesses: chronic fatigue syndrome, fibromyalgia, Gulf War syndrome, arthritis.

Neomycin and Streptomycin – antibiotics incorporated into vaccines, such as MMR (measles, mumps, rubella), Polio, Chickenpox (Varivax).

MSG or mono sodium glutamate – a neurotoxin, harmful to the brain and nervous system is used as a preservative in products such as the FluMist, intranasal influenza vaccine.

Milk proteins in some vaccines are the asthma/allergy connection. They can overload a potentially allergic child with enough allergens to induce asthma.[5]

Contaminated and foreign mediums may be used to cultivate vaccines. These are derived from dog kidney, monkey kidney, chicken and duck egg protein, chick embryo, calf serum and pig or horse blood and injected directly into our bloodstreams without the benefit of being filtered by our livers or digestive systems. We don't really know how the body really reacts to these foreign proteins. This has never been studied.

Other Reasons NOT to Vaccinate

- The fact that most of these vaccines contain multiple preservatives and toxins implies that they are unstable and unreliable without them.
- A high rate of adverse vaccine reactions is being ignored and denied by conventional medicine. Only about one-tenth of vaccine reactions are actually reported, because most go unnoticed.[6]
- There are no control group studies proving that vaccines are safe and effective.

- Many vaccines are contaminated with other bacteria and viruses, especially from chickens.[7]

> **New Survey in California and Oregon finds:**
> **Vaccinated Children 2 ½ Times More Likely to Have Neurological Disorders Like ADHD and Autism** http://generationrescue.org 06/26/2007
>
> A survey conducted by phone compared 17,000 vaccinated and unvaccinated children in 9 counties in Oregon and California. Among more than 9,000 boys age 4-17, the survey found vaccinated boys were 2 ½ times (155%) more like to have neurological disorders compared to their unvaccinated peers. Vaccinated boys were 224% more likely to have ADHD and 61% more likely to have autism.
>
> Percentages were higher in the older age bracket of 11-17. Vaccinated boys were 158% more likely to have a neurological disorder, 317% more likely to have ADHD and 112% more likely to have autism.
>
> Although the phone survey isn't perfect, the numbers point to the need for a comprehensive national study to gather critical information. For more details about the survey go to http://generationrescue.org/survey.html

DTaP or DPT Vaccine

DPT, DTP, DTaP vaccines address the diphtheria, tetanus and pertussis. DTaP stands for diphtheria, tetanus and acellular pertussis which are supposedly safer than its predecessor, DTP or DPT shot. Neurological side effects are, however, still being reported. It should be noted that the chronic dysfunctions associated with DPT followed a serious acute neurologic illness that occurred in children within 7 days after receiving it.[8]

Studies have shown that the DTP shot increases the incidence of bronchial asthma, allergic rhinitis and atopic dermatitis.[9,10]

MMR Vaccine (Measles, Mumps, Rubella)

Entire chapters and books have been written, covering the controversy about this vaccine. The controversy exists because many children have been damaged by this vaccine and people are speaking out. One such person is Dr. Andrew Wakefield, medical doctor and world expert on the topic. He has written many articles on the harmful effects of the MMR, including development of autism in biologically vulnerable children. He has made a great impact and, subsequently, there is an ongoing scientific investigation into Dr. Wakefield's research.[11,12]

Many other reactions to the MMR vaccine have been reported. They range from mild to severe: otitis media (ear infections), allergies, skin rashes, encephalopathy, convulsions, seizures and anaphylactic shock.[13] This is one of the vaccines parents are most fearful of.

Dangers Following Vaccines Received Simultaneously

Evidence of serious health consequences for infants, following simultaneously received vaccinations, was recently confirmed in the Journal of Pediatrics. Blood levels of CRP or C-reactive protein were measured after vaccination. CRP, short for C-reactive protein, is a blood marker indicating a heightened state of inflammation throughout the body.[14]

Serious Inflammation, Breathing Problems, Post Multiple Vaccines

"Cardio-respiratory Complications and C-Reactive Protein Responses Associated with Administration of Single and Multiple Separate Vaccines Simultaneously, " Pourcyrous, M., et al. *Journal of Pediatrics*, Vol 151, Issue 2, Pages 167 - 172 M.

Two or more vaccines were given the same day to 239 premature infants. A separate group of infants were given one shot at a time, every three days. The vaccines administered were DTaP, Hib, polio [IPV], hepatitis B and Prevnar. The findings were disturbing:

1) Very high CRP occurred in 85 percent of infants who received simultaneous vaccines and nearly 70 percent of infants who received the shots one at a time.
2) Gastro-esophageal reflux (GERD) and severe intra-ventricular hemorrhage (bleeding in the brain) occurred in infants who received vaccines simultaneously.
3) Cardio-respiratory events (stopped breathing) occurred in 16 percent of **all** infants within 48 hours after receiving the vaccines.
4) Infants who received DTaP, Prevnar and Hib as single injections experienced the largest number of cardio-respiratory events overall.

We can deduce from this study that when injected with multiple vaccines on the same day, the body induces the state of inflammation. This is actually a protective mechanism. However, when left unaddressed, it can cause inflammatory responses or illnesses, such as asthma, reflux and cardio-respiratory events.

One such disease is Type 1 diabetes. It was found in a study of 62 children, who were part of the Diabetes Autoimmunity Study, that when infants and young children have an elevated CRP level, they have an increased risk of developing Type 1 (insulin-dependent) diabetes in childhood.[15]

Serious Questions about Gardasil, the HPV Vaccine for Girls

Serious questions have emerged in the U.S. and Australia over Gardasil (the HPV Vaccine.) Three deaths and thousands of side effects have been reported following injection with this vaccine, which is now recommended for all pre-adolescent girls, for prevention of cervical cancer caused by the Human Papilloma Virus.

Keep in mind that:

1) it does not prevent all strains of the HPV virus and

2) it is causing serious health problems.[16]

Studies have revealed that the vaccine has caused severe headaches, dizziness, temporary loss of vision, slurred speech, fainting, involuntary contraction of limbs (seizures), muscle weakness, tingling and numbness in the hands and feet, and joint pain. Some of the girls have lost consciousness during what appears to be seizures. Reports were filed through the FDA's vaccine adverse event reporting system.[17,18] Gardasil also contains 225 mcg of aluminum, a metal that is potentially toxic to the nervous system.[19]

Parents, students and young adult women, ask yourselves: Do the risks outweigh the benefits? Is there really a benefit, since the vaccine doesn't prevent from all strains of HPV -- and cervical cancer is not a prevalent disease? *Do I really want to take this chance and impair my health?*

The Flu Shot or Nasal Spray

Many people think they are doing something smart and preventative by receiving the influenza vaccine – a flu shot or FluMist nasal spray. But, they can have serious repercussions. To begin with, they are both a chemical soup, made of various toxic ingredients. Some contain mercury (Thimerosal) or polysorbate 80, toxic preservatives. Some contain monosodium glutamate and formaldehyde. This is just the beginning.

Children, ages 5 and up, teens and adults, under 50 are targets of the FluMist. It is very easy to administer. And – no pain. However, side effects reported have been headaches, muscle aches, irritability and fever over 100 degrees. These are the very symptoms the vaccine is supposed to prevent.

Think of this as well. There is a thin protective bone at the top of the nasal passages. The olfactory (smell) nerves pass through this bone and line the nasal passages. They carry molecules to the brain that identify certain smells we are familiar with. This is a long-time recognized direct pathway to the brain. The down side is that intranasal injection of certain viruses may result in brain infection or inflammation. The virus can be carried to the brain.

Another issue is that of multiple viruses. Several patients of mine over the last 3 years have reported incidence of shingles or herpes outbreaks in the months following their influenza vaccine. At first, I found this to be more than coincidental, but made no accusations. Then, after at least 3 reports, I realized what the problem was. The "viral load" in the body was just too much for the immune system to handle. And so, it broke down.

In other words, when you have a virus, such as the chicken pox or herpes virus lying dormant, as so many of us do, and you inhale or are injected with another virus, the load on the body is more than you can handle. This is especially true during stressful times when the immune system has been depleted. So, the vaccine becomes the stimulus for the breakdown of the immune system.

The point I'm making here is that we are told to avoid getting a flu vaccine if we have a current infection. How would you know? You may have an infection with no symptoms. Or you may have a viral overload that you do not feel.

A person is also supposed to avoid taking a flu vaccine if they're on steroids (because they suppress the immune system). Asthmatics, Crohn's and arthritis patients often take steroids. For example, many inhalers are steroid-based.

In fact, a large percent of our population would by this definition, be considered immuno-suppressed. People in this category also have to avoid being around those who've received the FluMist vaccine. The virus in the vaccine can shed and be transferred through nasal fluid and saliva. Since nasal congestion and runny nose is the most prevalent side effect, this can be very dangerous. Think of restaurants, churches and other public facilities. Someone who has received the FluMist vaccine could sneeze near you or your food and if you're susceptible you could get very sick. The possibilities are endless.

Who Should NOT Receive the Flu Shot or Nasal Spray

- People who have had a severe reaction to a vaccination in the past
- Children less than 6 months old
- Pregnant women
- People who developed Guillain-Barre syndrome (GBS)
- People who have a severe **allergy to eggs**

Isn't it ironic that the elderly, the chronically ill and children between the ages of 6 and 23 months are the ones most susceptible to repercussions from the flu shots, yet they are put first in line when there is a shortage? In other words, when people have under-developed or compromised immune systems, flu shots and vaccines may be more toxic or damaging to them. For more flu shot information, see www.Safeminds.org.

10 Questions to Ask Before You Vaccinate

1. Do children under the age of 2 really need to be vaccinated at such a vulnerable age?
2. Does my child have a personal or family history of vaccine reactions, convulsions, neurological disorders, severe allergies, auto-immune or other immune system disorders?
3. Is my child sick right now? If so, should we wait to vaccinate when he or she is healthy?
4. How safe is the vaccine that is available? Look at both sides of this question. Don't just ask your doctor. Of course he or she is going to say that it's safe. That's their training – their belief system. Check the websites listed at the end of this chapter for the other side to this story.
5. What are the number and types of vaccines to be given simultaneously?
6. Do I have full information on the vaccine's side effects and ingredients?
7. Is the immunity provided by the vaccine solid and long-lasting?
8. How strong is the possibility that my child might contract the disease he/she is being immunized for?
9. What are the health consequences of the natural infection if contracted?
10. Are there alternatives to immunization that are they safe and effective?

How to Recognize Signs of Vaccine Reactions

With the increased number of vaccines given to young children, the probability of a child having a reaction is greater than ever. Many children receive 48 doses of 14 vaccines before the age of six.[20] This is a tremendous assault on a young body with an under-developed immune system.

A wide range of reactions are listed below. Some reactions are dramatic and others may go unnoticed because they could happen any day:

- Flu-like symptoms
- High fever
- Headaches
- Screaming
- Convulsions – shaking, twitching, trembling

- Seizures
- Brain inflammation - often starts with arching of the back and screaming
- Rash or hives
- Throat swelling
- Joint pain
- Shock or collapse
- Intestinal obstruction
- Behavioral changes: child can't sleep or refuses to eat
- Anaphylaxis - a sudden, severe, potentially fatal, systemic allergic reaction involving the skin, lungs, GI tract and cardiovascular system
- Sudden Infant Death Syndrome (aka SIDS, crib or cot death)
- Developmental disorders (autism, seizures, mental retardation, hyperactivity, dyslexia)
- Immune deficiency (e.g. Epstein Barr Virus, chronic fatigue syndrome, recurrent infections)
- Degenerative disease (e.g. muscular dystrophy, multiple sclerosis, arthritis, cancer, leukemia, lupus, fibromyalgia)

Toxic Metals from Vaccinations May Cause

- ADD/ADHD
- Allergies
- Autism
- Behavior problems
- Depression
- Developmental delays
- Digestive problems
- Hyperactivity
- Inability to handle stress
- Insomnia
- Learning disabilities
- Mood swings
- Nightmares
- Respiratory illnesses
- Seizures
- Unexplained fears

What If I Decide to Vaccinate or If My Child Has Already Been Vaccinated?

Building natural immunity is vital for all children, vaccinated or not. Certainly, building the immune system is important, before or after a vaccination. This may help the body rid the toxins from the vaccines more readily. Your child will still have other natural infections in life and the stronger the "internal army", the less problematic the infections will be.

There are protocols and modalities for vaccine detoxification, healing from vaccine injury and immune system strengthening. The best type of program is customized for your child's needs. Ask your health practitioner to help with this.

If your child has already been vaccinated, you should have them tested for toxic metals. Check *Chapter 5 on Toxic Metals* for further suggestions.

Minimize or Prevent Harmful Reactions to Vaccines

- Insist upon full disclosure of vaccine ingredients from your pediatrician. Research the ingredients and make sure you feel comfortable using these vaccines for your child.
- Use Thimerosal-free or mercury-free vaccines.
- Don't vaccinate ill children; their immune systems are already compromised.
- Do not give live viral vaccines to immunologically-challenged kids.
- Don't give multiple vaccinations in one visit. For instance, split out MMR vaccines by taking each – measles, mumps and rubella, separately. A new study advises that the MMRV vaccine, including varicella, be given individually. With the addition of the varicella, more children had seizures.[21]
- Avoid the MMR vaccine if the child is allergic to eggs.
- Avoid the Hepatitis B vaccine if the child is allergic to yeast.
- Don't administer the flu shot with other vaccines.
- Use immune-boosting supplements before and after vaccinations, such as Vitamin C, acidophilus, antioxidants such as glutathione, plant sterols such as Moducare and blue green algae.
- Eliminate sugar a few days before the vaccination, as it suppresses the immune system. Eat as purely and organically as possible.
- Make sure your child is structurally and functionally strong. Visit your chiropractor or osteopath periodically to ensure there is no interference with the nervous system that could suppress immune function.
- Check for toxic and heavy metals if your child has been vaccinated. Use hair analysis, urine-challenge testing or stool testing for toxic metals.
- Embark on a toxin or metal elimination program. (Consult with your natural health practitioner for an appropriate program.)

Recommendations vs. Laws

You can obtain affidavits for vaccine exemption – philosophical, medical or religious. Know the legal requirements of the vaccination laws in your State. Understand the difference between a legal requirement and a recommendation. For instance, while vaccine policymakers in the American Academy of Pediatrics (AAP) and the Centers for Disease Control (CDC) recommend that the MMR shot be given to all children, your State may legally require only measles and rubella vaccines. In this case, you have the legal option to vaccinate with only measles and rubella vaccines and not with mumps vaccine.

The National Vaccine Information Center (www.NVIC.org) is dedicated to disseminating information about vaccines and infectious diseases in order to prevent vaccine injuries and deaths through public education. They also defend the informed consent ethic. Their website is chock full of parent-friendly information that can help in the decision-making process, as well as hands-on tools for dealing with your state, your schools and other parents.

For school admission, most all States allow for medical exemption and religious exemption. Many allow for philosophical exemption. Check the Resource List at the back of book for further information.

---

1. *www.NVIC.org*
2. *Merriam-Webster Online Medical Dictionary, 2007*
3. *www.NVIC.com*
4. *"Addressing Parents' Concerns: Do Vaccines Contain Harmful Preservatives, Adjuvants, Additives, or Residuals?" Paul A. Offit, MD* and Rita K. Jew, PharmD, Journal of Pediatrics, Vol. 112 No. 6 December 2003, pp. 1394-1397*
5. *Archives of Pediatrics and Adolescent Medicine 1998 August;152:734-738*
6. *www.NVIC.com*
7. *Smallpox Vaccine: Does it Work? By Randall Neustaedter OMD, LAc, CCH, 07/18/2004, www.hpakids.org.*
8. *"DPT Vaccine Chronic Nervous System Dysfunction: A New Analysis (1994). Inst of Medicine, a division of the National Academy of Sciences*
9. *Archives of Pediatrics and Adolescent Medicine 1998 August;152:734-738*
10. *Pediatric Allergy and Immunology, Volume 19, Number 1, February 2008 , pp. 46-52(7)*
11. *Wakefield AJ. Enterocolitis, autism and measles virus. Molecular Psychiatry. 2002;7 Suppl 2:S44-46*
12. *"We won't allow MMR cover-up say parents of tragic toddlers", author Sue Corrigan, Daily Mail, UK, Sunday, 18th June 2006*
13. *http://www.nvic.org/Diseases/mmr.htm*
14. *Pourcyrous, M., et al. Primary Immunization of Premature Infants with Gestational Age Less Than 35 Weeks: Cardiorespiratory Complications and C-Reactive Protein Responses Associated with Administration of Single and Multiple Separate Vaccines Simultaneously. Journal of Pediatrics, Volume 151, Issue 2, Pages 167 - 172 M.*
15. *Chase HP, et al. Elevated C-reactive protein levels in the development of type 1 diabetes. Diabetes. 2004 Oct; 53(10):2569-73.*

16. *"Questions over human papillomavirus vaccine in the US and Australia", Tanne, Janice, British Medical Journal, June 9, 2007;334:1182-1183, doi:10.1136/bmj.39237.424537.4E*
17. *Merck & Co., Inc. 2006. Gardasil product insert: Serious Adverse Experiences.*
18. *Food and Drug Administration. May 18, 2006. FDA Background Document for Vaccines and Related Biological Products Advisory Committee: Gardasil. Table 32.*
19. *Food and Drug Administration. May 18, 2006. FDA Background Document for Vaccines and Related Biological Products Advisory Committee: Gardasil HPV Quadrivalent Vaccine.*
20. *www.NVIC.org*
21. *"Guidelines Update for Administration of Combination MMRV Vaccine", Morbidity and Mortality Weekly Report, Mar 14, 2008; 57:258-260.*

~ ~ ~

Chapter Seven

The Rx Generation

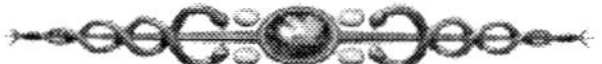

This is the era of fast solutions. Go to the doctor, get the drug, get back on your feet, and move on. When we take our children to the pediatrician, the fast solution is the drug. Now, that is what doctors do – prescribe drugs. It's expected; it's their training.

We, in today's world, take our children to their pediatrician multiple times per year. What used to be a once-a-year formality, has become a monthly necessity. Whether it's for an ear infection, asthma, ADD or depression, prescription drugs are routine for children today – and sometimes they are used for years on end. And, we are educating our children that we need drugs to help us feel better.

Indeed, some parents and families, as well as teachers are relieved that their child or student is on medication. In the cases of ADD or ADHD, the child has become more compliant or focused. As a health practitioner, I have seen both the up and down sides of medications.

But, if you're walking into your living room and the curtains are on fire because your son wanted to burn down the house, then maybe the medication that controls his behavior is a good idea. Extremely stressful family situations may warrant drug use, at least as a stopgap measure -- until their lives get back on track. But, could it be that in most cases, we are …

Too Quick to Drug Our Children?

Our children are in danger and the statistics are staggering. Children are now second only to senior citizens, as the fastest growing group of prescription drug-takers. A new study has found that children are spending 34 percent more of their time - more of their life -- on medications.[1]

So, kids are spending more time on medications and families are spending more dollars. In a 2004 analysis of 300,000 children under the age of 19, the following was determined:[2]

The Cost of Over-Prescribing ADHD drugs

- From 1997 to 2002, spending on prescription medicines for pediatric patients rose 85%.

- Spending on prescription drugs for ADHD increased 122% from 1998 to 2002.
- For children under the age of 19 years, spending for prescription drugs grew 28% last year. This is the highest percentage of growth among all age groups.
- Most startling was the 369% increase in spending on ADHD drugs for kids under the age of five.

A Staggering Increase in the Use of Other Pediatric Meds

- Use of antidepressants for children increased 21%.
- Use of medicines for autism and other conduct disorders jumped 71%.
- Use of gastrointestinal drugs, including those for babies with colic, rose 28%.[3]

These mind-blowing figures represent a dangerous state of affairs. The incidence of children using prescription drugs has skyrocketed because the diagnoses of mental and physical illnesses have skyrocketed. The diagnoses have increased because that is what happens when you go to most doctors. You go in the box and get the drug.

Some experts are concerned that increased prescribing is due to over-diagnosis or unnecessary diagnosis. Others believe that children today are just plain sicker now than in previous times. We also see how aggressive pharmaceutical companies are in marketing their products. This is all true. The problem is that many parents think that taking a drug is normal. It is common, but not normal – and certainly not healthy. We have lost our focus on the potential of the body to bring itself into balance. We have forgotten our knowledge about the healing power of food and nutrients. We are busy; we are uninformed. That's just the way it is. But have no fear; the "grass roots" is here. There is a change in the air. Some people are becoming more proactive, more independently-minded – one by one. Let's get the facts under our belts.

THE CULPRITS

The Stimulants: AD/HD Meds

This is the biggest scandal and the most malicious issue in the industry of children's health. Millions of children are on anti-psychotic medications. Two- and three-year olds are being assessed by psychiatrists for ADHD, bipolar disorder, depression, violent behavior and insomnia. All the docs know how to do is prescribe meds. They haven't been taught about the options. The parents are the ones who initiate and seek out the alternatives. Someone has to.

Stimulant drugs are the most commonly prescribed psychiatric drugs for children.[4] Many of these medications are being used "off label", which means there are no studies, no science to back up their safety. They are unapproved. This is a crime. Who knows what damage is being done to the body – nervous system, kidneys and liver. What about behavioral side effects? There are no long-term studies to assess this. Then, when the medication stops working, another is prescribed --- sometimes three or four at once.

In 1995, the International Narcotics Control Board stated that 10 to 12 percent of all boys between the ages of 6 and 14 in the United States had been diagnosed with ADD and were routinely treated with (Ritalin) methylphenidate. Their findings: "For the most widely medicated childhood condition, Attention Deficit Disorder, there is no current, validated diagnostic test."[5] Can you believe it? And about 90 percent of global consumption is in the United States.[6] Yet, with all the warnings and no validating studies, Ritalin and its "cousins" continue to be prescribed, more and more.

Ritalin was the first ADHD drug to use methylphenidate, a stimulant, as its active ingredient. Today, Ritalin has been replaced with the drugs Stratera, Adderall, Concerta or Metadate. Stratera is not a stimulant drug, but the others are. Adderall's active ingredient is amphetamine and Concerta and Metadate contain the same stimulant as Ritalin – methylphenidate. The difference is they are time-released, in hopes of causing less appetite suppression and less disruptive sleep.

Who besides parents and concerned health professionals are looking at the problems these drugs cause and alternatives to their use? Dr. Peter Breggin, psychiatrist, states in his book, *Talking Back to Ritalin*, that Ritalin disrupts a child's growth hormones, cardiovascular system, digestive system, brain chemistry and central nervous system.[7]

The following studies reinforce what you may be feeling in your gut – that these medications can be not only unhealthy, but dangerous.

Psychostimulants Cause Toxicity of the Central Nervous System (CNS)

"Psychostimulants in the treatment of children diagnosed with ADHD: Risks and Mechanism of Action", Breggin, Peter R., Director, International Center for the Study of Psychiatry and Psychology (ICSPP), *International Journal of Risk & Safety in Medicine 12* (1999) 3–35 3, IOS Press

This report states, "Psycho-stimulants produce a continuum of toxicity based on ...CNS excitation with direct effects on various neurotransmitter systems, including dopamine, norepinephrine and serotonin. The continuum begins with feelings of increased energy, hyper-alertness. It progresses toward insomnia, obsessive/compulsive or preservative activities, agitation, hypomania, mania, and sometimes seizures."

Other adverse drug reactions are nervousness, irritability, anxiety, depression, and increased emotional sensitivity or easy crying. Occasionally, they can cause impaired cognitive performance, compulsions, decreased social interest, and, in the extreme, a "zombie-like" feeling.

Ritalin Use and Potential Cancer Risk

"Cytogenetic effects in children treated with methylphenidate" Randa A. El-Zein, RA, Abdel-Rahman, SZ, Hay, MJ, Lopez, MS, Bondy, ML, Morris, DL, Legator, MS, *Cancer Letters*, Volume 230, Issue 2, 18 December 2005, Pages 284-291.

Preliminary research points to Ritalin posing potential health risks, such as increased risk of cancer. All participants in this study had chromosomal abnormalities after being on Ritalin for three months. These initial findings warrant further investigations.

19 Sudden Deaths in Children Treated with ADHD Drugs

"Heart test urged before kids get ADHD drugs: Stimulants can leave some vulnerable to cardiac arrest, heart group says", MSNBC News, April 21, 2008

An FDA review revealed report of 19 sudden deaths in children treated with ADHD drugs and 26 reports of other problems including strokes and fast heart rates between 1999 and 2003.

Stimulant drugs, like Ritalin, Adderall and Concerta, can increase blood pressure and heart rate. Because children with heart conditions may be vulnerable to sudden cardiac arrest, the American Heart Association recommends that children should be screened for heart problems before getting drugs that treat hyperactivity and attention-deficit disorder.

"A Prospective Study of Delinquency in 110 Adolescent Boys with Attention Deficit Disorder and 88 Normal Adolescent Boys,"

J. Satterfield, et al, *American Journal of Psychiatry*, June 1982, p. 6.

"These findings suggest a strong relationship between childhood ADD and later arrests for delinquent behavior...our study is consistent with other follow-up studies of <u>drug-treated</u> children that have found an <u>absence</u> of long-term beneficial effect..."

"Panel: ADHD Drugs for Kids Need Hallucination Warning"
Rubin, Rita, *USA TODAY*, Mar 22, 2006

According to a report in the March 22, 2006 issue of USA Today, "a Food and Drug Administration advisory committee recommended ...that the agency add information about a possible risk of hallucinations in children to the labels of attention deficit/hyperactivity disorder drugs."

The FDA was urged to develop a Medication Guide explaining to parents that certain risks might accompany taking ADHD medications - Adderall, Focalin, Concerta, Metadate, Methylin, Ritalin and Dexedrine. In addition to increased risk of hallucinations, other risks may be heart attack, stroke or sudden death in patients who have undiagnosed heart problems.

The panel decided against using a "black box" warning for these risks, as they thought that would scare parents away from the drugs. One such drug, however, Stratera, does carry a "black box" warning about risk of suicide.

In addition to the "side effects" and dangers stated in the above studies, substance abuse can also be the consequence of taking daily stimulant or amphetamine-like medications. A child, teen or young adult can develop a higher tolerance for a drug and need to take more to get the same "high" or the same effects. This is due to damage or loss of the receptors of the brain chemical, dopamine, and can lead to intense cravings and alcohol or other addictions.

When you combine substance abuse with hallucinations, toxicity, cancer and death, you get powerful reasons to avoid use of stimulant drugs for your children. There are alternatives that work. Many of them are in the following chapters of this book.

Abuse of Stimulant Medications on the Street

Schedule II drugs, such as Ritalin, Adderall and Concerta have a high degree of abuse-potential just like all amphetamine-based products. After all, cocaine and morphine are also Schedule II drugs. A report from the National Center on Addiction and Substance Abuse indicates that there has been a 93 percent increase in the abuse of ADHD drugs for enhanced studying and test-taking. High school and college students purchase Adderall and Ritalin on the street; they crush and snort them to stay awake and alert.[8] The after-effects are devastating: headaches, anxiety, depression, high blood pressure and possible stroke.[9]

Lawsuits and ADD Medication

Several class action lawsuits have been brought against manufacturers of ADD and ADHD medications. They have all been dismissed before they went to trial. One lawsuit charged that Novartis (manufacturer of Ritalin) conspired with the American Psychiatric Association to promote more drug sales by "creating ADD".[10] ADD and ADHD are real, they are not made up. They are however, over-exaggerated, and as we know, the conventional medical world does not know how to treat "the person" – just the symptom. If you create a name for a problem, it is easier to prescribe a drug for the solution.

Review

In summary, there are several concerns in the medical community about medication use for ADHD:

1. A rise in occurrence of ADD and ADHD among children in the last 20 years
2. Classification of our children as having mental illnesses
3. Increased use of prescription drugs for "treatment" of ADD and ADHD
4. Increased spending on stimulant drugs
5. Probability of damage to heart, the brain chemistry, metabolism and the hormones of children on stimulant medications

For further information on the use of drugs for children diagnosed with ADD or ADHD look at the works of Dr. Peter Breggin (breggin.com), Jon Rappoport (nomorefakenews.com), and Dr. Lawrence Diller (docdiller.com).

Anti-Depressant and Anti-Anxiety Medications

Medication use for depression in children rose 21 percent between 1997 and 2002.[11]

Most of the drugs prescribed for children and adults with depression are called SSRI's or Selective Serotonin Reuptake Inhibitors. These drugs are designed to manipulate the brain chemical, serotonin, which is a mood elevator and anti-depressant that the body manufactures.

Prozac, Zoloft and Paxil are SSRI anti-depressants. They carry a long list of side effects, including insomnia, headache and nervousness. Major depression is sometimes treated with tricyclic anti-depressants such as Tofranil and Norpramin, but they are not common anymore. They also attempt to normalize the brain chemicals or neurotransmitters.

Medications for anxiety work in a similar way. In fact, many antidepressants like Celexa, Lexapro, Luvox, Paxil, Prozac and Zoloft are commonly prescribed to treat the symptoms of anxiety. Other drugs, such as Klonopin and Xanax, known as benzodiazepines, are also used for anxiety disorders. About 13 percent of children between 9 and 17 years old have an anxiety disorder.

Girls are affected more than boys.[12] This means they have fear, scary thoughts and perceive danger. Anxiety is also characterized by feelings of persistent, uncontrollable worry over an extended period of time. Significant distress may be seen in various areas of a child's life: school, peer relationships, social gatherings, home and travel away from home. It may cause panic, nervousness, compulsiveness or insomnia – and certainly can limit a child's ability to engage in a variety of normal activities.

The following studies reveal serious concerns with children using anti-anxiety and anti-depressant medications.

Anti-depressant Drug Therapy and Suicide in Severely Depressed Children and Adults, Olfson, M, MD, MPH; Marcus, SC, PhD; Shaffer, D, MD, *Archives of General Psychiatry*. 2006; 63:865-872.

A case-controlled study of 5,500 adults and children has revealed that many commonly used anti-depressants may increase suicide risk for children and adolescents, especially those who are severely depressed.

These drugs are Celexa, Paxil, Prozac and Zoloft. Children aged 6 to 18 were 1.5 times more likely to attempt suicide and 15 times more like to die from the attempt, than children who were diagnosed as depressed, but not treated with drugs. The risk was increased with children treated with one of these drugs for the first time and post hospitalization.
Effexor, a serotonin-norepinephrine re-uptake inhibitor (SNRI) was associated with 2.3 times the risk of suicide attempts. The anti-depressant manufacturers have therefore been advised to add a warning on these drug labels in a special black box, making health care providers aware of the risk.

Cover-Up: Paxil Linked to Teenage Suicide
"Secrets of the Drug Trials", BBC, January 29, 2007

In a BBC report in January of 2007, drug maker, GlaxoSmithKline was exposed for skewing and distorting clinical trials with Paxil (or Seroxat in the United Kingdom). The company claimed that the drug was useful in treating children with depression, but apparently Paxil failed in the clinical trials. Information was revealed that teenagers taking the anti-depressant had increased risk of suicide. Among other toxic side effects were tendency toward hostility and violence. Bereaved families are now taking legal action.

(You wonder if the reason drugs are called by different names in other countries, is for damage control.)

What is most disturbing is the growing list of children and teenagers who have gone on violent rampages – some on school grounds. The wake-up call came in 1999 with the Columbine school shooting, but there were many before and many following that horrendous incident. One common denominator in many of the school shootings is that the shooter had been diagnosed with a mental disease and was on anti-depressant or anti-anxiety medication.

In the provocative report, *Why Did They Do It*? Jon Rappoport, investigative reporter raises many points about violence in children and teens. In some of the school shootings, the offenders or the shooters had been treated for depression, ADD or anxiety and had a history of use of prescription drugs like Prozac, Ritalin, Luvox and others.[13] He also calls attention to the fact that the media downplays or excludes this information from its articles and reports.

The question is -- did drugs tip these children and teens over the edge? Did the young shooters have nutritional deficiencies, hormonal imbalances and toxic drug effects?

There must be some explanation. Yes, there's a change in parenting, a need for classroom and school reform, too much TV and too many video games. But there is a missing link here.

One connection most scientists and doctors are not making is – the body and the brain work together. And often times, there is a physical or physiological cause underlying cognitive, emotional and behavioral problems. We discuss these causes in *Chapter 8.*

Bi Polar Disorder and Multiple Medications

Bi Polar disorder or manic-depression in children has risen considerably in the past ten years. It is characterized by mood changes that go in cycles. There are periods of severe highs or mania and severe lows or depression, with normal moods occurring between cycles. Mood swings typically follow each other very closely, within hours or days. Sometimes they are separated by months to years. These "highs" and "lows" can vary in intensity and severity.

There has been a tremendous increase in the diagnosis of bipolar disorder in children. Likewise, the use of medications to treat it has risen. As seen in the following exposé, this diagnosis often overlaps with others:

The "New Syndrome": Bi Polar Disorder
"The Medicated Child", Frontline, January 8, 2008, www.pbs.org/frontline/medicatedchild

"The number of American children identified as bipolar is now over a million and rising."

More Bi Polar is diagnosed in the US than any other country. Bi-polar is characterized by temper tantrums, explosive irritability and drastic mood swings.
It's probably a syndrome and that's one reason that kids with Bi Polar Disorder are often on more than one medication. Bi Polar overlaps with ADHD and Obsessive Compulsive Disorder.

As stated above, many children with bipolar disorder are taking more than one medication. What some experts have noticed is that children on ADD or ADHD medications for a period of time eventually become diagnosed as bipolar. Could the AD/HD medications possibly be causing bipolar tendencies? It is common that while most children start on one medication, eventually another is added as the original benefit seems to "wear out".

When bi polar does co-exist with AD/HD, psychiatrists may prescribe mood stabilizers, anti-psychotics, benzodiazepines or other medications along with their AD/HD medications. Many of these children and adolescents are at particular risk for substance abuse, as well as health problems and emotional imbalances resulting from overlapping medications that have not been tested for their compatibility.

Greed may have also fueled this explosion in the frequency of diagnosis and the use of medications for bipolar disorder. A New York Times article in June of 2008 exposed a group of psychiatrists at the Harvard Medical School who failed to disclose earnings from pharmaceutical companies for research. In other words, they had a conflict of interest. The Harvard group's consulting arrangements with drug makers were already controversial because of the researchers' advocacy of unapproved uses of psychiatric medicines in children. The controversial 40-fold increase from 1994 to 2003 in the diagnosis of pediatric bipolar disorder has been attributed to <u>this</u> Harvard group.[14]

Pay particular attention to the stacking of medications if your child is diagnosed as bipolar. Ask a lot of questions. An additional disease added to your child's list may be required because the prior drug has lost its effectiveness. These drugs change the brain chemistry and can cause other imbalances. Bipolar disease may be nothing more than a "side effect" of AD/HD medication. For more information on biochemical and nutritional causes, see *Chapter 8.*

Rise in Children Using Prescribed Sleep Medications

Insomnia, not being able to fall asleep or stay asleep, is a concern for many children today. About 10% of parents in the U.S. think their child has a sleep problem.[15] Many of them are treated with prescription drugs, such as anti-histamines, benzodiazepines, anti-depressants and sleep medications. The Food and Drug Administration, however, has not approved most of these drugs for childhood sleep problems:

Unapproved Prescription Drugs for Childhood Sleep Problems

"Trends in Medication Prescribing for Pediatric Sleep Difficulties in US Outpatient Settings" Stojanovski, SD, Rasu, RS, Balkrishnan, R, Nahata, MC, Sleep. 2007 Aug 1; 30 (8):1013-7 17702271.

81% of the children seen by their doctor for sleep problems resulted in prescriptions for medication. "Many of these medications were frequently used to treat children with sleep difficulties ... despite lack of FDA approved labeling to assure their effectiveness and safety in this population", said Dr. Nahata, who conducted the study on patients 17 years of age and younger with sleep difficulties from 1993-2004.

Only 7% of the children were advised to receive dietary counseling and 22% were prescribed behavioral therapy, such as psychotherapy and stress management to relieve the sleep problems.[16]

The majority of children in the above study were between 6 and 12 years of age. Why are they not sleeping; why are they sleep-walking; why are they snoring? Here are just a few logical answers:

- caffeine intake in colas and sports drinks
- excess sugar and dairy consumption
- hyper-stimulating food additives
- video game anxiety
- nutrient-deficient fast foods

Eliminate all of the above, and most sleep problems will improve. Why do we skip right to the drug solution, before trying dietary and other behavior modification?

Psychiatric Drugs and Young Children

Another matter that is unforgivable is the use of prescribed drugs for young children. Researchers reported an astronomical increase in the use of psychiatric drugs among 2 to 4-year olds in three regions of the U.S. This study, in the *Journal of American Medical Association* in 2000, reviewed more than 200,000 preschool-age children between 1991 and 1995. The number of children taking Ritalin and other stimulants increased 200 percent and those taking anti-depressants like Prozac, increased 150 percent.[17]

Experts say they are troubled by the findings, because the effects of such drugs in children so young are largely unknown. Some doctors worry that such powerful drugs could be dangerous for a child's development. Dr. Joseph T. Coyle of Harvard Medical School's psychiatry department said the study reveals a troubling trend, "*Given that there is no empirical evidence to support psychotropic drug treatment in very young children, there are valid concerns that such treatment could have deleterious effects on the developing brain.*"[18] Consider that 90 percent of total brain growth occurs within the first three years of life.

The number of young children getting any of the drugs totaled about 100,000 in 1991, and jumped 50 percent to 150,000 in 1995. That year, 60 percent of the youngsters on drugs were age 4, 30 percent were age 3 and 10 percent were 2-year-olds.[19]

"The Perils of Pills"

"The Psychiatric Medication of Children is Dangerously Haphazard", Shute, N, Locy, T and Pasternak, D, Cover Story, *U.S. News & World Report*, March 2000.

"According to the U.S. Surgeon General, almost 21% of children age 9 and up have a mental disorder, including depression, ADHD and bipolar disorder."[20] Robert Johnson, director of adolescent medicine for the University of Medicine and Dentistry of New Jersey said, "We know more about the effects of marijuana on kids than Prozac." "There's all risk and very little benefit for the ...two drugs (Prozac and Clonidine)", says Steven Hyman, Director of the *National Institute of Mental Health.*

Errors in Prescribing Pediatric Medications

The FDA estimates that more than half of the drugs approved every year are inadequately tested and labeled for use in pediatric patients. The majority of drugs prescribed for pediatric use do not have FDA approval for pediatric use.[21]This means that they are used "off label". It also leaves a lot of room for mistakes to be made in the calculation of milligrams and doses for newborns and young children. Average doses are established for adults, not necessarily children.

The range is wide for variations in age and weight and a serious mistake could be made in so much as the misplacement of a decimal point. A recent survey has shown that orders for pediatric patients often contain problems relating to poor handwriting, misused abbreviations, decimals and poor calculations. In a review of 200 medication-related errors, more than 50 percent of errors found were attributed to decimal placement, calculations of the dosage.[22]

Most importantly, children are not just small adults. They are more fragile, with under-developed detoxification systems. Their absorption, metabolism and elimination of the drugs changes considerably as they mature. The pharmacokinetic properties must be aligned with these changes.[23,24]

The liver and especially the kidneys have less ability to clear drugs from the system and can incur life-threatening damage, the younger a child is. While the liver reaches adult capacity to metabolize drugs in about six months or more, the kidneys take over a year to reach this maturation.[25] In summary, improperly prescribed drugs for infants and young children can result in liver or renal failure.

Think twice – or more – before you decide to give your child a prescription drug. Double check with your doctor about the appropriate dosage.

Anti-Histamines, Anti-Inflammatories

The incidence of asthma and allergies has doubled in the past 25 years. It is estimated that 7 percent of all children are asthmatic and 25 percent have allergies.[26] The use of asthma medications jumped 15% from 2000 to 2003.[27] Asthma and allergies affect the lungs and respiratory tract. Our children are being denied a most basic right - the right to breathe - the right to live without the fear of losing their breath.

Steroid medications and inhalers have become essential for controlling breathing in some children. They can have, however, damaging effects on the adrenal glands, the stress-balancing organs. No wonder so many kids have difficulty handling stress and adapting to change. No wonder they have mood swings, depression, energy problems, hyperactivity and diminished cognitive function. Their adrenal stress hormones, cortisol, DHEA and adrenalin have been affected. These hormones can be checked through saliva testing and the adrenals can be fortified naturally, if imbalance occurs. (See section on Hormone Imbalance in the next chapter.)

Our adrenal glands carry us through all the phases of our lives, helping us adapt to change and to deal with trauma and loss, joy or pain. These glands are intimately connected with the nervous system, so they affect our emotions and behaviors. They are the key to stress-relief and balance. They also manufacture the sex hormones: estrogen, progesterone and testosterone. Premature hormonal development may result, saddling some children with both severe physical and emotional challenges.

DO NOT under-estimate the impact that most prescription medications have on our adrenal glands. This is an UNLISTED side effect. We become more susceptible to illness and stress, and we pre-maturely age when our adrenal glands become unbalanced.

Cough Medications or Speed?

They seem so innocent – the cough medications in most families' medicine cabinets. After all, they are available over-the-counter and who hasn't used them? Well, the label warnings on these products, about consulting your doctor before giving them to young children, are there for a reason: they contain potentially dangerous ingredients.

DM or dextromethorphan is an ingredient in many cough medicines that has been linked to neurological damage in children. In addition, decongestants that contain pseudoephedrine, can cause heart arrhythmias and increase blood pressure in some children. If this doesn't give you reason enough to avoid them, the chemical soup of synthetic dyes, flavorings and artificial sweeteners are toxic and can exacerbate symptoms of ADHD.

A harmless alternative for soothing a cough is honey and lemon juice; it is simple, effective and there are no label warnings.[28]

Antibiotics Top the List

Antibiotics still top the list of most commonly prescribed drugs for children. It's time for us and our doctors to end the love affair with them. Antibiotics are over-prescribed and used unnecessarily because they are the only tools in the toolbox and because they provide a simple answer for a patient who doesn't know any different.

Here's the problem. Many children have been on 5, 10, 20 rounds of antibiotics for ear infections, sinus, throat and respiratory infections, before they are even 10 years old. These are toxic drugs that contain harmful chemicals. A quick fix can turn into a chronic disease down the road – asthma, digestive disturbances, eczema, liver and kidney dysfunction.[29]

Research shows that this common practice is not even justified for many respiratory, throat and ear infections.[30] Several studies indicate little to no benefit of antibiotic use for these infections and more risk than they're worth.[31]

Also, in many instances, infections are viral in nature and antibiotics only have activity against bacteria. So, here, they are worthless.

Furthermore, antibiotic resistance is becoming one of the world's most pressing health problems. This occurs when bacteria mutate or change in some way that reduces the effectiveness of the drug. Widespread inappropriate antibiotic use is fueling this problem.[32] As bacteria become more resistant, infections become tougher to treat.

Let's give our kids' bodies what they need to defend themselves. Why wait to be attacked. We can strengthen our immune systems to protect us. Bacteria are all around. We mustn't succumb. We are not weak. Our children need to know that they are strong, that they can defend themselves without relying on drugs. Reserve the antibiotics for life-saving necessities. This is where they shine, not in day-to-day life.

Summarizing all there is to know about medications for children is a formidable task. There is so much more to learn. For further information about this topic, especially about medications for attention and behavior problems see these books:

Toxic Psychiatry: A Psychiatrist Exposes the Dangers of Mood-Altering Drugs
by Peter Breggin, M.D.

The Ritalin Fact Book:
What Your Doctor Won't Tell You About ADHD and Stimulant Drugs
by Peter Breggin, M.D.

The Antidepressant Fact Book:
What Your Doctor Won't Tell You About Prozac, Zoloft, Paxil, Celexa and Luvox
by Peter Breggin, M.D.

Talking Back to Ritalin: What Doctors Aren't Telling You About Stimulants and ADHD
by Peter Breggin, M.D.

The Last Normal Child: Essays on the Intersection of Kids, Culture, and Psychiatric Drugs
by Lawrence H. Diller, M.D.

Should I Medicate My Child? Sane Solutions for Troubled Kids with--and without--Psychiatric Drugs by Lawrence Diller, M.D.

Running on Ritalin: A Physician Reflects on Children, Society, and Performance in a Pill
by Lawrence H. Diller, M.D.

***The Survival Guide for Kids with ADD or ADHD* (Kid-friendly tools to make each day a great one.)**
No young ADD'er should miss the book 'Signs That Tell You Medicine Is Working.'
by John F. Taylor, Ph.D.

Helping Your Hyperactive ADD Child
by John F. Taylor, PhD

Driven To Distraction: Recognizing and Coping with Attention Deficit Disorder from Childhood Through Adulthood
by Edward M. Hallowell and John J. Ratey

Why Can't My Child Behave? Why Can't She Cope? Why Can't He Learn?
by Jane Hersey and Robert C. Lawlor

"Why Did They Do It: An Inquiry into the School Shootings in America,"
by Jon Rappoport, Position Paper #1, The Truth Seeker Foundation (www.nomorefakenews.com)

---

1. *http://www.cbsnews.com/stories/2004/05/17/health/main617768.shtml, Kids' Behavior Drug Use Soars: Spending for Medicines Passes Antibiotics, Asthma Drugs, May 17, 2004. (based on a survey by Medco Health Solutions, Dr. Robert Epstein. The Associated Press contributed to this report.)*
2. *IBID*
3. *IBID*
4. *"Trends in Psychotropic Medication Costs for Children and Adolescents, 1997-2000", Martin A, Leslie D, Archives of Pediatrics and Adolescent Medicine. 2003;157(10):997-1004*
5. *"Dramatic Increase in Methylphenidate Consumption in US: Marketing Methods Questioned", International Narcotics Control Board Annual Report, 1995, United Nation's Information Service Press Release, 28 February 1996*
6. *IBID*

7. *Breggin, PR, Talking Back to Ritalin: What Doctors Aren't Telling You About Stimulants for Children, 1998.*
8. *"Dramatic Increase in Methylphenidate Consumption in US: Marketing Methods Questioned", International Narcotics Control Board Annual Report, 1995, United Nation's Information Service Press Release, 28 February 1996*
9. *Pure Facts, the newsletter of the Feingold Association of the United States, November 2007, www.feingold.org.*
10. *Class Action Reporter Newsletter, co-published by Bankruptcy Creditors' Service, Inc., Princeton, NJ, and Beard Group, Inc., Washington, DC. Theresa Cheuk, Managing Editor, May 2001 http://bankrupt.com/CAR_Public/010430.MBX*
11. *http://www.cbsnews.com/stories/2004/05/17/health/main617768.shtml, Kids' Behavior Drug Use Soars: Spending for Medicines Passes Antibiotics, Asthma Drugs, May 17, 2004. (based on a survey by Medco Health Solutions, Dr. Robert Epstein. The Associated Press contributed to this report.)*
12. *U.S. Surgeon General Report on Mental Health, Children and Mental Health, Chapter 3, 1999, http://www.surgeongeneral.gov/library/mentalhealth/chapter3/sec1.html.*
13. *Rappoport, J, Why Did They Do It? An Inquiry into the School Shootings in America, The Truth Seeker Foundation, 1999*
14. *"Child Experts Fail to Reveal Full Drug Pay", Harris, G and Carey, B, New York Times, June 8, 2008.*
15. *National Sleep Foundation Poll, 2004, www.sleepfoundation.org.*
16. *"Trends in medication prescribing for pediatric sleep difficulties in US outpatient settings", Sasko D Stojanovski, Rafia S Rasu , Rajesh Balkrishnan , Milap C Nahata, Sleep. 2007 Aug 1; 30 (8):1013-7 17702271.*
17. *Zito JM, Safer DJ, dosReis S, et al: "Trends in the prescribing of psychotropic medication to preschoolers", Journal of American Medical Association, 283:1025-1030, 2000.*
18. *Coyle JT: "Psychotropic drug use in very young children", Journal of American Medical Association, 283:1059-1060, 2000.*
19. *IBID*
20. *Nancy Shute, Toni Locy and Douglas Pasternak, "The Perils of Pills", U.S. News &World Report, cover story, March 6, 2000 (http://www.usnews.com/usnews/culture/articles/000306/archive_021339.htm)*
21. *"Pediatric Dosing Considerations", Ellen Whipple Guthrie, and PharmD, US Pharm. 2005; 12: HS-5-HS-10.*
22. *"Challenges in Pediatric Pharmacotherapy: Minimizing Medication Errors", from Medscape Pharmacists, Amy L. Mitchell, PharmD, http://www.medscape.com/viewarticle/421220*
23. *Blaho K, Winbery S, Merigian K. Pharmacological considerations for the pediatric patient. Optom Clin . 1996; 5:61-90.*

24. *Ginsberg G, Hattis D, Miller R, Sonawane B. Pediatric pharmacokinetic data: implications for environmental risk assessment for children. Pediatrics. 2004; 113(4 suppl); 973-983.*
25. *Koda-Kimble MA, Young LY. Applied Therapeutics: The Clinical Use of Drugs. 5th ed. Vancouver, WA: Lippincott Williams & Wilkins; 1992.*
26. *http://www.cbsnews.com/stories/2004/05/17/health/main617768.shtml, Kids' Behavior Drug Use Soars: Spending for Medicines Passes Antibiotics, Asthma Drugs, May 17, 2004. (based on a survey by Medco Health Solutions, Dr. Robert Epstein. The Associated Press contributed to this report.)*
27. *IBID*
28. *Pure Facts, the newsletter of the Feingold Association of the United States, November 2007, www.feingold.org.*
29. *"The Risk of the Hemolytic–Uremic Syndrome after Antibiotic Treatment of Escherichia coli O157:H7 Infections", Tarr, PI, M.D., Wong, CS, M.D, et al, New England Journal of Medicine, June 29, 2000, Volume 342:1930-1936, No.26*
30. *"Antibiotics Not Justified for Respiratory Tract Infections, Sore Throat, or Otitis Media", News Author: Barclay, L, MD, and CME Author: Charles Vega, MD, Online First Issue of the British Medical Journal, October 18, 2007.*
31. *IBID*
32. *http://www.cdc.gov/Features/GetSmart/*

~ ~ ~

Chapter Eight

HOW PHYSICAL CONDITIONS AFFECT BEHAVIOR and EMOTIONS

"The body says what words cannot."

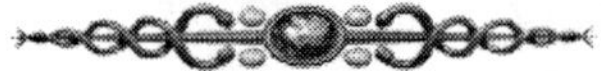

Emotional and Behavioral Problems Linked to Physical Imbalances?
"Mental Health in the United States: Health Care and Well Being of Children With Chronic Emotional, Behavioral, or Developmental Problems", Journal of American Medical Assoc, Nov 2005; 294:2567-2569.

Two thirds of the participating children with emotional, behavioral and developmental problems also had chronic physical conditions, such as asthma, allergies, diabetes, frequent headaches, hearing or vision problems, or bone, joint or muscle problems.

The study above is a good example of the body-mind connection. It makes sense that people with chronic emotional and behavioral problems would also have certain physical symptoms. In the ideal world, we would address the physical, mental and emotional problems simultaneously. But in this age of defined specialties, we seem to lose perspective on wholeness. Physical symptoms are overlooked as unrelated to the emotional or behavioral, and vice versa.

In other words, headaches are treated with aspirin or Tylenol, and not linked to the child's behavior or ADHD. Depression is treated with an anti-depressant, and not considered a result of low blood sugar or stress hormone imbalance.

These physical symptoms are clues to both the cause and the treatment of many mental and emotional disorders. They are not isolated during a traditional medical diagnosis. But if they were discovered through other forms of testing, then they could be addressed. And we would begin to see a lessening of the mental, emotional and behavioral problems. In fact, a whole new world would be revealed.

In this world, the brain and the physical body talk to each other. We are a great bundle of energy with billions of communicating electrical transmissions –

not a shell with disjointed organ systems. Most conventional doctors make diagnoses that are going to affect a child for years to come, with no tests and no correlations to physical body. They don't seem to see the connection between the brain and the body of their patients – the people sitting right in front of them. What a slip-up; what an oversight.

Parents see this connection more than the doctors do. They see and know their child as a whole person, who by the sheer definition of a human being has a body and brain that work in tandem. They dance, they flow, or they have two left feet.

By identifying the underlying physical connections to the mental, emotional or behavioral problems and addressing them with specific super foods, homeopathics and nutritionals, the whole child emerges – the one you know – deep down inside.

Here are the eight major nutritional and biochemical imbalances related to mental, emotional, behavior and learning problems:

1. Blood Sugar Imbalances
2. Nutrient Deficiencies
3. Infection
4. Allergies and Sensitivities
5. Toxicity or "Body Overload"
6. Metabolic Imbalances
7. Hormone Imbalances
8. Neurotransmitter Imbalances

1. Blood Sugar Imbalance

Blood sugar imbalance is one of the main contributors to cognitive, behavioral and emotional disorders among children. High or low, blood sugar imbalance is often undiagnosed. Therefore, it is not considered to be a medical problem. But it is a nutritional problem and it can lead to serious disruptions in brain chemistry, stress hormone regulation and metabolism.

Most blood sugar imbalances in children are in the low-blood-sugar realm, such as hypoglycemia. However, there is a greater incidence today of high blood sugar, insulin resistance and diabetes than ever before. Let's examine each one:

Low Blood Sugar - Hypoglycemia

Low blood sugar is prevalent among children with symptoms of ADD, ADHD, dyslexia, learning problems and autism, as well as those with mental disorders: schizophrenia, manic depression, bi-polar disorder and clinical depression. Some behaviors characteristic of hypoglycemia are mood swings, "acting out", erratic behavior, "foggy" thinking, indecision and "dreaminess". These can be caused by over-eating refined and white flour carbohydrates, sugars, sodas, fruit drinks and nutrient-depleted food. In other words, these foods have empty calories. They do not provide the nutrients and quality of fuel needed for sustained energy for the body or the brain.

The biological explanation is that refined and sugar foods cause a swift release of insulin from the pancreas. This results in a speedy delivery of glucose to the brain and muscles, creating an energy surge or "high". However, when glucose leaves the bloodstream so fast, the body "crashes" with a "low". Such is the balance of nature. These "lows" are experienced as fatigue, headaches, and cravings. Hyperactivity, irritability, grumpiness, depression and inattention may also result. This "roller coaster" activity can cause a child to be unpredictable, flighty, unstable and unhappy.

I had a boyfriend who would hallucinate that he was sitting above his car as he was driving. This was after eating half a loaf of bread. Thankfully, he began to put two and two together, that he had low blood sugar. He worked on balancing his blood sugar naturally. If he had not figured this out, I'm sure he would be on some kind of medication right now --- probably for depression or bi-polar disorder. The mind is a crazy thing. It can go into so many crevasses – some happy, some not, especially when it is not fueled properly.

Insulin Resistance

Insulin resistance, sometimes called *dysglycemia* may develop if a person with hypoglycemia doesn't know they have it, or doesn't learn how to control it. So, insulin resistance or *dysglycemia* result from poor blood sugar management. They are the first step toward diabetes.

Here is a stepwise description of the process:

A. When we eat grains, fruits, bread, cereal, pasta, rice, desserts, sweet drinks, alcohol and sugar, the pancreas makes insulin to help deliver the glucose or sugar from the bloodstream to our body and brain cells for fuel and energy. Insulin is a hormone that acts like a key, opening the door of the cells to let the glucose in. This is a normal process.

B. Overuse of carbohydrate and sugar foods causes this process to escalate. Excess insulin is then produced.

C. Over time, the body's cells become "bombarded" with excess insulin.

D. Insulin flooding the cells causes stress on the body and the cells become less responsive to insulin. In other words, they become resistant to the insulin. They close their doors. Normal amounts of insulin are then, inadequate to produce a normal insulin response from fat, muscle and liver cells.

E. This insulin resistance in fat cells causes triglyceride levels to elevate in the blood. Triglycerides are stored there.

F. Insulin resistance in the liver reduces glucose storage, causing higher glucose in the blood and lowered energy and endurance for the individual.

G. High plasma levels of insulin and glucose due to insulin resistance often lead to metabolic syndrome and type 2 diabetes.

The biggest factor contributing to these imbalances is the amount of refined carbohydrates a person eats. The American Diabetes Association estimates that 41 million people in the U.S. are pre-diabetic; many of them are children and teens. In fact, one in six overweight teenagers between ages 12-19 are pre-diabetic.[1]

It is estimated that the average American eats 158 pounds of sugar each year. This places an enormous strain on the pancreas and its ability to secrete insulin, to control glucose levels. Resultant symptoms of insulin resistance are weight gain, high cholesterol and triglycerides, mood swings, inability to store magnesium, muscle pain, fatigue, brain fog, learning disabilities, anxiety and depression.

In 2000, a study in *Diabetes Care* revealed that overweight children with high levels of insulin in their blood were also likely to have high levels of homocysteine, a substance which can raise the risk of heart disease and stroke.[2] It is amazing that this all results from overeating refined carbohydrates and sugar -- something very preventable. The following chart shows the progression of blood sugar conditions:

The Dance of Glucose and Insulin

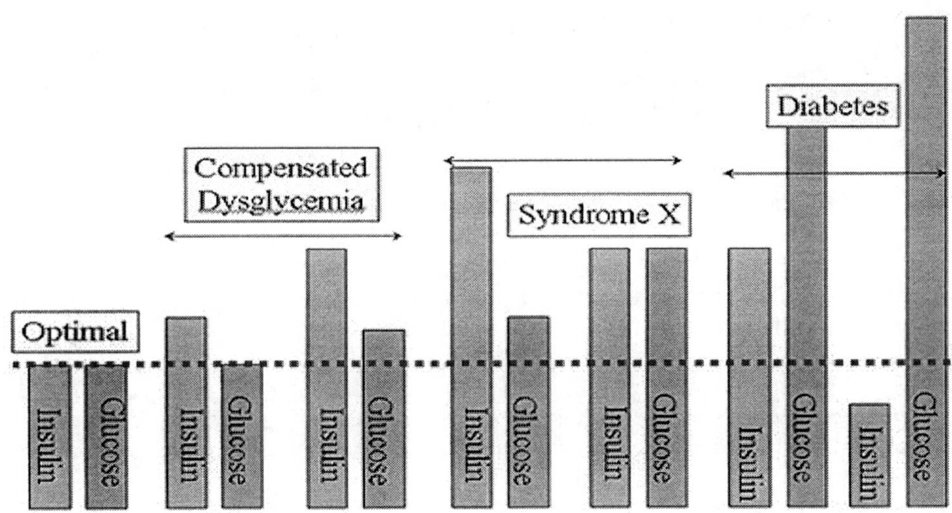

Everyone should aim for being in the optimal range, with both optimal glucose and insulin levels. Since insulin is a storage hormone, a person usually stores body fat and this is seen – yes – in the gut, the stomach area. When this happens, people are sometimes called “apple-shaped”.

Next, cholesterol and triglycerides (blood fats) levels often rise in the blood. This can be determined with a lipid panel blood test. Because the cells reject or resist the insulin, glucose levels begin to rise.
So, prolonged insulin resistance can cause:

- depression
- fatigue
- focus & concentration issues
- heart disease
- high blood pressure
- high cholesterol
- high LDL
- high triglycerides
- inflammation
- low HDL
- obesity
- pain
- polycystic ovary syndrome
- thyroid problems

Syndrome X or Metabolic Syndrome

Syndrome X is the next stage after insulin resistance. People are labeled with Syndrome X when they have a cluster of symptoms or conditions encompassing high cholesterol, high triglycerides or high blood pressure. Weight loss is very difficult at this stage, as insulin levels become very high and uncontrollable, leading to fat storage. This is the step before Type 2 diabetes; it is reversible.

Hyper-insulinism or Hyper-insulinemia

This refers to a higher-than-average level of insulin in the blood, as related to blood glucose. Hyperinsulinism can exist with both low and high blood sugar.

Diabetes

Diabetes is a chronic disease in which the body does not make or properly use insulin, the hormone needed to convert glucose and other food into energy. With insufficient insulin, the glucose in the blood builds up or rises and spills into the urine. As a result, the body loses its main source of fuel. There are two types of diabetes:

Type 1 diabetes
Type 2 diabetes

Type 1 Diabetes

Juvenile diabetes or Type 1 diabetes is on the rise. It is an autoimmune disease in which the immune system destroys the insulin-producing beta cells of the pancreas that regulate blood glucose. Since the pancreas can no longer produce insulin, children and adults with type 1 diabetes require daily injections of insulin for life. They are at risk for long-term complications such as damage to cardiovascular system, kidneys, eyes, nerves, blood vessels, gums and teeth.

Type 1 diabetes accounts for 5 to 10 percent of all diagnosed cases of diabetes. A plan for managing diabetes includes insulin therapy, self-monitoring of blood glucose with a glucometer, healthy eating and regular physical activity.

Healthy eating means in-taking the nutrients that are important for keeping the blood sugar balanced. Mom's nutrition during pregnancy is also very important. This is why prenatal vitamins were designed – to insure that all nutritional bases are covered. And this focus must be continued throughout breastfeeding and/or formula-feeding. Unfortunately, many children become malnourished from inadequate or poorly absorbed nutrients in their infant formula. For instance, research shows that intake of vitamin D during infancy may help prevent diabetes.

Vitamin D May Help Prevent Type 1 Diabetes in Children
Zipitis CS and Akobeng AK, "Vitamin D supplementation in early childhood and risk of type 1 diabetes: A systematic review and meta-analysis", *Arch Dis Child* 2008 Mar 13; [e-pub ahead of print]. (http://dx.doi.org/10.1136/adc.2007.128579)

An analysis of several European studies indicates that supplementation with vitamin D between ages 7 and 12 months, was associated with a lowered risk of type 1 diabetes. One form of vitamin D used was cod liver oil.

Type 2 Diabetes

After insulin resistance progresses, type 2 diabetes can develop. In time, the pancreas can not keep up with the demands for insulin production so insulin levels decrease and blood glucose levels rise even more. Type-2 diabetes is no longer just for grown-ups, and that is the sad truth, according to the U.S. News magazine. Experts at the Centers for Disease Control say that about 1 in 50 children have type 2 diabetes and the numbers are increasing.
This condition used to be called adult onset diabetes because it was so rare in children. But type 2 diabetes is now seen in teens and young children, even as young as 3 and 4 years old.[3] A CDC study estimated that 1 in 3 children born in 2000 will develop diabetes in their lifetime.[4]

Epidemic of Type 2 Diabetes in Youth
"Glucose and Insulin Metabolism in Obese Youth", Burgert, TS, *Pediatric Endocrinology Review*, 2006 Dec; 3 Suppl 4:555-5594.

Pediatricians are concerned about the health implications, as the prevalence of childhood obesity increases. Most striking is the unprecedented epidemic of abnormal glucose metabolism, with the diagnosis of type 2 diabetes outnumbering the diagnosis of type 1 diabetes mellitus in many pediatric endocrine clinics.

There are serious implications here. The younger the children are when they develop type 2 diabetes, the younger they are going to develop complications with other body organs. For instance, we are going to see more young adults with type 2 diabetes developing serious kidney problems, heart attacks and blindness. An enormous burden of responsibility and self-care is put on these children.

Obesity and overweight are issues with 90 percent of the children with type 2 diabetes. Couple their sedentary lifestyle with the poor quality food, especially sugar, sodas and snack foods, and you have a formula for this degenerative illness.

Parents of children who are obese or overweight should pay particular attention to the child's energy level -- is he or she often fatigued? Observe his or her emotions – are there mood swings? How do they sleep? Nightmares? Do they urinate a lot or are they excessively thirsty? These are all symptoms that may point to diabetes. This is especially true for those children who have a parent or other relative with this condition.

Type 2 diabetes is not difficult to control. Weight loss, exercise and a glycemic-controlled diet can be the answer here. This "diet" requires an awareness of what foods cause blood sugar imbalances and therefore an insulin response. It involves avoiding high-glycemic carbohydrates, like sugar, and replacing them with low and medium-glycemic carbohydrates, such as fruits and vegetables. (See *Chapter 11 on Special Diets*)

Hands down, we as a society eat a high glycemic diet -- fruit juice, cereal with sugar or pancakes with syrup in the morning; white bread or pizza, fruit juice or soda for lunch; a piece of fruit, candy bar, more fruit juice for a snack; and white bread on the burger, soda or more fruit juice, or macaroni and cheese for dinner; then there's dessert. No wonder we are overweight, hypoglycemic and diabetic.

And the children are at the greatest risk, because many of them started from day one with sugar in their infant formula. We are addicted and it's not O.K. Sure, there is a special place for high-glycemic carbohydrates and sugar. Social eating, celebrations and splurges are a fact of life. Everyone likes to have fun with food. But high-glycemic foods are for special occasions, not daily fare. The study below represents the fact that whole grains and protein foods are more stabilizing for the blood sugar than refined flour foods:

Overeating results from eating high glycemic foods

Ludwig, DS, et al, "High Glycemic Index Foods, Overeating, and Obesity", *Journal of Pediatrics*, Vol. 103, No. 3, March 1999, p. e26.

In this study, adolescents who ate processed instant oatmeal for breakfast ate more food later in the day than those who were fed unprocessed oatmeal. Instant oatmeal has a higher ***glycemic index***. It is digested and absorbed more rapidly. Too rapidly. High-glycemic index foods induce hormonal changes that lead to decreased availability of metabolic fuels, excessive hunger, and overeating in obese subjects.

This study suggests dietary advantages for treatment of obesity: 1) high quantities of vegetables, legumes and fruits, 2) a decrease in using high-glycemic carbohydrates, and 3) a moderate amount of protein and fats.

Moreover, reducing high-glycemic foods can positively affect cholesterol and triglyceride levels and risk of diabetes mellitus.

Below are dietary suggestions for balancing your child's blood sugar:

1. Eat high nutrient foods -- vegetables and fruits.
2. Eat high fiber foods: raw fruits and vegetables, legumes, whole grains.
3. Eat a low-glycemic diet (see *Special Diets Chapter 11*).
4. Eat 4-5 small meals throughout the day, evenly spaced.
5. Eliminate hydrogenated fats and oils and utilize good fats (*Chapter 2*).

2. Nutrient Deficiencies

Vitamins, Minerals, Essential Fatty Acids, Amino Acids

Nutrient deficiencies are so simple to correct, yet very common. They arise when our children eat nutrient-depleted, processed and fast foods. Inefficient digestion and absorption also contributes to vitamin, mineral and other nutrient deficiencies. This is, in essence, a form of malnutrition and has its repercussions: poor focus, concentration and memory, mood imbalances, susceptibility to infections of the sinuses, ears, lungs and skin, damaged metabolism, and stunted growth and development.

Most nutrient deficiencies go unnoticed by your pediatrician, so you have to be a nutrition detective in order to discover them. It is not so difficult. After you read this book, you'll know more than many medical experts on the topic. B vitamin deficiencies are probably the most common among the vitamins nowadays. The B vitamins are necessary for balancing stress: physical, mental and emotional. So energy production, blood sugar balance, mood stabilization and good cognitive function require a balance of the B's, especially B5, B6 and B12.

Vitamin C is also important for stress balancing, as well as immune system strength. It may be deficient in children who don't eat enough fruits and vegetables.

The fat-soluble vitamins, A, E and K may be less likely deficient, however vitamin D deficiency has become more common since children don't play outside very much anymore. This occurs especially in the winter, when children are less likely to be soaking up the sun. The sun helps the body manufacture vitamin D. A great source of both vitamins A and D is cod liver oil.
The two most common mineral deficiencies among children are magnesium and zinc. These minerals are required for balanced brain and nervous system functions. (See the *Chapter 13* for more information.)

Additionally, the electrolyte minerals, sodium, potassium and chloride, are nutrients that constantly "get used up" and need replacing. They "ignite" electrical activities in the body and brain, cellular energy, respiration, kidney and heart function.

Electrolyte deficiencies cause dehydration and this is much more complex than just being thirsty or not drinking enough water. Stress is put on many organs when the electrolytes become unbalanced: kidneys, heart, skin, brain, GI tract and potentially every cell of the body. The following are the most common symptoms of dehydration:

- confusion
- dizziness
- dry mouth and tongue
- dry mouth, mucous membranes
- dry skin
- fatigue
- high fever
- increased heart rate & breathing
- irritability
- less frequent diaper-wetting
- less frequent urination
- light-headedness
- listlessness
- no tears when crying
- skin that does not flatten when pinched & released
- sunken belly, eyes or cheeks
- thirst

Causes of Dehydration

- a hyper-acidic body
- caffeine intake
- diarrhea
- excess sugar consumption
- excess sweating
- high fevers
- intake of carbonated drinks
- lack of water intake
- mineral deficiencies
- stress
- use of antihistamines
- use of diuretics
- use of laxatives
- use of steroids
- use of stimulant medications
- vomiting

Any of the above dehydration symptoms can render the body mineral deficient. Using a good electrolyte mineral supplement can be very helpful. Most people think of Pedialyte, but there are much higher quality products that you can obtain from your health practitioner or your health food store, such as Spectra Min (Energetix), Rehydration (Energetix) or EmergenC (Alacer).

The Body's Storehouse

We are robbing our children's banks. When the body needs to produce certain chemicals for metabolism or for neurotransmission (brain chemistry), it needs vitamins and minerals to do so. It needs the essential fatty acids or good fats and the essential amino acids or proteins to do so. If they are not taken in from the food, the body will rob its own nutrient banks, its storehouses, such as muscles or bones - in order to make what it needs. Otherwise, the proper body or brain chemicals will not be manufactured.

This has devastating effects down the road. We have a designated storehouse of nutrients that we draw upon when we need to – for stressful situations. But if the storehouse is robbed during youth and perpetually, then we are not be able to physically and mentally, handle stressful events when they arise. If you keep withdrawing from the bank account without re-depositing, funds are unavailable.

Just one example of the consequence of nutrient depletion may be seen in the amount of crime and violence we have in our society today. The following study is indicative of how replenishing deficient nutrients can positively change a person's life:

A Government's Secret Weapon in Fighting Crime: Healthy Eating

Gesch, BC, et al, "Influence of supplementary vitamins, minerals and essential fatty acids on the antisocial behavior of young adult prisoners," *The British Journal of Psychiatry* (2002) 181: 22-28.

This double-blind, placebo-controlled study is one of the first to show a scientific link between healthy eating and crime. In a British prison, half the prisoners of all ages and ethnic backgrounds were given vitamins, minerals and essential fatty acids. The other half received a placebo.

--The group that took the supplements committed 25% fewer offences.

--The greatest reduction was for serious offences, including violence which fell by 40%.

--There was no such reduction for those on the placebo.

Conclusion: Antisocial behavior and violence in prisons are reduced by vitamins, minerals and essential fatty acids with similar implications for those eating poor diets in the community.

Cravings and Addictions (Is there a method behind the madness?)

Love of certain foods is one thing that makes the world go 'round. We all have our desires – the foods that make our tongues hang out. Unnatural food cravings however, appear as obsessions. They can lead to a distorted perception of food and even eating disorders. When children crave certain foods, there is often a reason – a reason based on body needs -- nutrient deficiencies:

- **Sugar:** need for brain fuel, such as amino acids and minerals; need for body fuel or energy; presence of infection or yeast in the body. They thrive on sugar.
- **Bread**, cereal, pasta: need for brain and body fuel; blood sugar may be out of balance; presence of infection or yeast in the body
- **Salt**: need for minerals for supporting the adrenal glands in producing energy; need for water or dehydration. The body craves salt to help retain water.
- **Cheese**: need for EFA's (essential fatty acids) for brain power; need for proteins/amino acids for proper neurotransmission and muscle fuel
- **Highly seasoned or spicy food**: need for nutrients, especially vitamins and minerals; zinc deficiency can lead to impaired sense of taste and smell. Some people require strong tasting food because they don't taste anything otherwise.
- **Ice**: need for iron, B12, folic acid. This may indicate anemia.
- **Dirt or clay**: need for minerals or other nutrients. People with the eating disorder, *pica*, crave non-food substances. The body is looking for nutrition from dirt, clay, soap, paint chips, cigarette ashes or broken crockery. Serious mineral deficiencies, as well as metal toxicity can lead to this disorder.

3. Infection

Infection sounds like an unusual cause for a cognitive, emotional or behavior problem. It doesn't surprise me when someone has a curious, scrunched-up look on their face when we discuss this topic.

The plain fact of the matter is that there are many underlying infections with children and adults. But a person may have no symptoms of infection, at least not outwardly. You don't have to have a cold or flu. It may be much more subtle, and in fact, much deeper than that.

Infections can be many and varied: bacterial, viral, yeast, fungal, or parasitic. Whenever I interview a parent about their child, I always start at the head and move down, body part by body part, to the feet. We cover the eyes, ears, nose, teeth, gums, throat, lymph nodes, skin, digestive tract, bowels, urination, body discomfort, pain, inflammation and so on. The link to infection is often revealed during this process.

One way to check for infection is to do a comprehensive stool panel, which can be ordered by your family doctor or your alternative family practitioner.

Many traditional stool tests do not reveal anything, so it is important to make sure you are ordering your test from a practitioner who uses a specialty lab, not a conventional medical or hospital lab. Recommended laboratories are Diagnos-Techs and Great Smokies Labs. Ask your practitioner or family doctor to insure that the lab checks for yeast, fungus, mold, bacteria, all types of parasites, gluten, casein, soy, egg, inflammatory markers and enzyme markers. Otherwise, you are probably wasting your time.

When the test results come in, make sure your doctor explains what they mean. There is a lot of information in these tests that can be glossed over if someone doesn't pay attention. It happens all the time. If a parasitic, bacterial or yeast infection is found, then you know what you're dealing with and can treat it or eradicate it. Your health practitioner may recommend natural anti-infective supplements such as citrus seed extract, olive leaf extract, cat's claw, echinacea, goldenseal, garlic, caprylic acid, wormwood oil, neem oil or oregano oil. Always incorporate probiotics like acidophilus and bifidus to enhance immune function at the same time.

So, infection can cause alterations in brain chemistry, effecting moods, behavior and cognitive function. The following study reveals fascinating new and old information about infection linked to some cases of psychosis:

Infection and Psychosis? "Are some cases of psychosis caused by microbial agents? A review of the evidence", R H Yolken and E F Torrey, *Molecular Psychiatry* (2008) 13, 470–479; doi:10.1038/mp.2008.5; published online 2-12-08

The infectious theory of psychosis, prominent early in the twentieth century, has recently received renewed scientific support. Evidence has accumulated that schizophrenia and bipolar disorder are complex diseases in which many predisposing genes interact with one or more environmental agents to cause symptoms.

The protozoan Toxoplasma gondii and cytomegalovirus are examples of infectious agents, linked to schizophrenia. The identification of infectious agents associated with the development of schizophrenia might lead to new methods for the diagnosis, treatment and prevention of this disorder.

Candida Albicans or Yeast

Candida albicans is a yeast-like organism that commonly grows in the body. It is normal to have some candida. We always have good and bad critters. They co-exist in the balance of nature. Overgrowth of this pathogen in the intestinal tract is however, not normal and can manifest in a variety of ways.

It can cause acne, skin rashes, constipation, diarrhea, gas, bloating, cramping, itching, thrush, ear infections, vaginal yeast infections, bladder infections, eczema, psoriasis, hives, sinusitis, asthma, parasitic infection and intense cravings for sugar, desserts, breads and fermented products.

If yeast overgrowth becomes systemic, throughout the body, mental and emotional symptoms such as foggy thinking, slow mental processes, attention deficits, hyperactivity, anger, frustration, depression, forgetfulness, hallucinations and mood swings may be exacerbated. Checking for yeast or candida overgrowth can be done through the home-collection stool testing that we mentioned above.

Antibiotics often cause yeast problems or infections. They kill the good bacteria while targeting the bad, and yeast overgrowth occurs because the good bacteria are not there to keep it under control. If your child has had antibiotics for ear infections, sinusitis, respiratory or other infections, there is a good chance that an abundance of yeast or other pathogens may occur in the body. **It is important to realize that antibiotics do not kill yeast. They make yeast thrive.** Other causes of yeast overgrowth are the overuse of sugar, refined white flour products, milk-drinking, prescription drugs, the birth control pill, tap water and alcohol.

The study below reveals an unusual manifestation of yeast overgrowth:

The "Auto-Brewery" Syndrome - Yeast Overgrowth

Abnormal Gut Fermentation: The "Auto-Brewery" Syndrome", Joneja, JM, Ph.D.; Ayre, EA, Ph.D.; Paterson, K, RDN; *Journal of the Canadian Dietetic Assoc,* Vol. 58, No. 2, Summer 1997

Yeast or bacterial fermentation in the small intestine is created by increased levels of blood ethanol from abnormal gut fermentation, and absorbed into the bloodstream.

A person may even act "drunk" as if he or she has consumed alcohol. This causes psychological, gastrointestinal, respiratory, and musculoskeletal problems. Due to malabsorption of nutrients, **deficiencies can result: B vitamin, zinc and magnesium.**

Common symptoms: abdominal discomfort, bloating, mucus discharge, aches and pains, intense cravings for sugar, behavior "as if you were drunk", hyperactivity, hard to wind down, hives, eczema, chronic vaginal yeast infections and addictive tendencies.

In addition to avoiding foods that cause yeast proliferation, there are a variety of nutritional supplements that can be taken to expedite the healing progress. Acidophilus and bifidus, the good bacteria, and digestive enzymes can very helpful. Powerful yeast killers are grapefruit seed extract, neem oil and wormwood oil. Tea tree oil and oil of oregano are also excellent.

4. Allergies and Sensitivities

Allergies are abnormal responses to an allergen (food or environmental substance) causing the immune system to react with inflammation or congestion. Sinusitis, otitis, eczema, skin rashes and difficulty breathing are just some examples. Allergic responses can make people feel uncomfortable and can cause pain. They are responsible for more visits to the doctor's office than any single disease in this country. The prevalence of allergies in today's world is astonishing:

- Allergies or "allergic disease" is the 3rd most common chronic disease among children under 18 years old.[5]
- In 2002, 14% or 9 million children had asthma. That's 25% higher than the year before.[6]
- Another 9 million children have respiratory allergies or hay fever.[7]
- Allergic rhinitis affects up to 40% of children.[8]
- On any given day, 10,000 American children miss school because of allergic rhinitis, for an annual total of 2 million lost school days.[9]
- Studies have shown that most people with asthma also have seasonal or perennial allergic rhinitis.[10] Rhinitis coexists in more than 75% of people with allergic asthma and in more than 80% of those with non-allergic asthma.[11]

Environmental allergens are the ones most commonly associated with asthma, rhinitis and seasonal allergies:

- animal dander
- automotive exhaust
- cosmetics
- drugs
- dust
- household chemicals
- industrial chemicals
- insect venoms
- mold
- paint fumes
- perfumes
- pollen

These allergens can be ingested, inhaled or contracted on the skin. Allergic symptoms, therefore, can take form in and affect many different organs and body tissues:

General: chronic fatigue, joint pain, muscle aches, arthritis

Head: headaches, drowsiness, hyperactivity, panic attacks, depression, learning disabilities, dyslexia

Nose: runny nose, sneezing, post nasal drip, recurrent sinusitis
Ears: ear infections, otitis, swollen glands, impaired hearing, dizziness, tinnitus
Skin: hives, rashes, eczema, dermatitis, pallor, psoriasis, itching, scaling
Eyes: redness, itching, swelling, tearing, blurred vision
Respiratory: asthma, wheezing, tightness in the chest, cough, recurrent bronchitis
Digestive tract: stomach ache, bloating, irritable bowel, constipation or diarrhea, colitis
Genital-Urinary tract: urinary tract symptoms, vulvadynia, chronic vaginitis, prostatitis

Though environmental allergies are the ones that first come to mind for most people, food allergies may be just as damaging, if not more. They are overlooked by many physicians. This is probably because they are a bit elusive, not always a black and white issue. You may not know you have them because you don't always feel them. They can actually make environmental and seasonal allergies worse.

The major allergy foods are:

- Chocolate
- Corn (on the cob, chips)
- Dairy (milk, cheese)
- Eggs
- Gluten-containing grains
- Oranges & other citrus fruits
- Peanuts
- Shellfish (shrimp, crab)
- Soy
- Strawberries
- Sugar
- Tomato (ketchup, sauces)
- Tree nuts (almond, walnuts)
- Wheat (bread, cake, bagels)

So, about peanuts. Though closely related, they are not really in the nut family; they are legumes. Many children with peanut allergies are very sensitive to peanuts or peanut products and can't even be in the same room as a peanut-containing food, or he/she will have a violent anaphylactic reaction. This could be life-threatening, causing constriction of the bronchi and difficulty breathing.

Some schools now have a separate peanut butter table in the cafeteria, for the kids with peanut butter sandwiches to sit at, and some schools have banned peanut butter from the school grounds altogether.

You may be asking yourself, "Why is this happening?" Why have peanut allergies more than tripled in the last five years? One reason is that peanut butter today is not what it used to be. It contains many more additives - sugar, hydrogenated fats and emulsifiers. Peanuts are also one of the most pesticide-ridden crops.

Now, with commercial peanut butter, we're getting additives, pesticides and – mold. Most peanuts also contain a carcinogenic mold called *aflatoxin.* And it turns out that many kids with mold allergies, such as asthmatics and those with eczema, are hyper-sensitive to commercial peanut butters because of this. Aflatoxin does not grow in dry climates, so peanuts from New Mexico, such as the Valencia peanuts used in the organic Arrowhead Mills brand are much safer. Other foods that may contain aflatoxin are pecans, pistachios, walnuts, grains, soybeans and spices.

Three Classifications of Food Allergies:

1. fixed
2. delayed
5. variable

1. Fixed allergy or "IgE" mediated food allergy - A person with a fixed food allergy reacts to that substance each time they come into contact with it, even if it's a tiny exposure. It doesn't matter how long it has been since the last exposure, re-exposure will still produce a reaction. This type of allergy is often inherited or genetically determined. These foods may need to be completely removed from the diet or avoided if symptoms are serious. In many cases, if you strengthen the immune system, the reaction will reduce.

2. Delayed, hidden, or IgG mediated food allergy - This is a cumulative type of allergy. The body develops antibodies against foods eaten frequently. This type of allergy is called food sensitivity and can create a chemical imbalance leading to digestive difficulties, gastric reflux, bowel problems, irritability, hyperactivity, depression, or pain.

Many chronic illnesses are triggered by food allergies which are delayed for up to three days. Since the reaction often goes unnoticed, it can cause chronic inflammation. Some conditions that result from IgG allergies or sensitivities are irritable bowel syndrome, Crohn's disease, lupus, multiple sclerosis and rheumatoid arthritis.

Common sensitivities are to foods containing chemicals, such as salicylates. (See Feingold information in *Special Diets Chapter 11.*) Many other foods have the potential to cause sensitivities, and the most common one is gluten, found in many grains. Others are casein in milk products, albumin in the whites of eggs and soy protein.

Celiac Disease - Gluten Sensitivity

This is generally a delayed and often hidden allergy or sensitivity, causing damage to the mucosal surface of the small intestine. It is a chronic digestive disorder, found in individuals who are genetically susceptible. Gluten, a protein in wheat, is the culprit.[12] It is also a component of durum, semolina, spelt, rye, barley, triticale and kamut.

When these gluten-containing grains are consumed, the absorptive villi, hair-like structures on the surface of the small intestine become damaged. This results in an inability of the body to absorb vitamins, minerals, carbohydrates, fats and proteins.

Astounding new numbers from a recent, large multi-center study indicate that one out of every 133 Americans has celiac disease and that thousands of people go undiagnosed each year. A person may not even be suspicious of having this condition because it is not necessary that they have any digestive difficulties in order to be diagnosed. That is why it slips through the cracks.[13]

It is estimated that only about 3% of the people who have celiac disease, know it. That means that 97% of them don't. The following conditions may be associated with gluten sensitivity:

- Bone disease and osteoporosis
- Central and peripheral nervous system disorders, due to nutrient deficiencies
- Pancreatic disease
- Intestinal cancers
- Other food sensitivities - to soy, egg, lactose, casein in dairy products
- Dermatitis, psoriasis, eczema
- Rheumatoid Arthritis
- Sjogren's Disease
- Systemic Lupus
- Diabetes Mellitus
- Depression
- Rheumatoid Arthritis
- Fibromyalgia
- Anxiety disorders
- Sensory Processing Disorder (SPD)

Common symptoms related to celiac disease and gluten sensitivity:

- abdominal cramping
- alternating constipation and diarrhea
- anemia

- bloating and abdominal distention
- bone or joint pain
- chronic constipation
- chronic diarrhea
- depression
- fatigue
- gas
- irritability
- short stature due to malabsorption[14]
- steatorrhea (foul smelling, floating stools)
- weakness
- weight loss due to malabsorption

Early Gluten-Free Diet May Prevent Autoimmune Diseases in Celiac Patients,
Journal of Pediatrics, August 2000; 137:263-265.

Studies reveal that people with celiac disease have high levels of diabetes- and thyroid-related auto-antibodies that "disappear" when the patients are placed on a gluten-free diet. 90 children with celiac disease were tested for serum antibodies to islet cells in the pancreas and cells of the thyroid. The prevalence of diabetes- and thyroid-related auto-antibodies was 11.1% and 14.4%, respectively.

The researchers then hypothesized that "a gluten-free diet started early may prevent other autoimmune diseases frequently associated with celiac disease." Scientists now suspect that gluten antibody dependency may affect people with other auto-immune disorders such as lupus and rheumatoid arthritis.

Another study in the *World Journal of Gastroenterology* in 2007 indicates a link between celiac disease and Hashimoto's thyroiditis.[15] People with high thyroid antibodies, may be able to normalize them by going gluten-free.

Is it also possible that the gluten molecule, so prevalent in today's diet, may affect those ***without*** celiac disease? People with other autoimmune diseases such as rheumatoid arthritis, multiple sclerosis, lupus and Sjogren's disease have experienced a decrease or elimination of symptoms after eliminating gluten. A percentage of these people may have celiac disease, but many may not. They may, however, be gluten sensitive. There are different levels of disease – different stages of development.

Other facts:

- Celiac disease can be activated anytime from infancy to adulthood
- Caucasians are mostly susceptible
- Most cases go undiagnosed
- You can do a saliva test for genetic gluten sensitivity. (www.enterolab.com)

The future of wheat and gluten grain consumption for people with celiac disease or gluten sensitivity is very individual. Some people benefit from eliminating gluten for six months to a year, healing the gut in the meantime and after challenge testing each grain, can add one or more back into their diets. Others, however, with more severe sensitivities can not use any gluten products.

This is not the end of the world. There are ample foods now on the market, in health food stores and through the internet that you can purchase to replace any gluten-containing product. (See *Chapter 2*.)

Finally, some people with celiac disease or gluten enteropathy have intestinal infections, especially parasitic. Once the infections are taken care of, the reaction to gluten diminishes or disappears altogether and the gut heals. This is a controversial area, but one certainly worth exploring with your health practitioner. The specialized stool testing described in *Chapter 3*, should be done to ascertain what infections may exist.

3. Variable food allergy – This is the most interesting, but complex type of allergy. A person may have a reaction to a food at one time, but not another. This can relate to pollen or mold allergy, but is a masked or hidden food allergy. For example:

a) In ragweed or hay fever season certain foods such as milk, melon or bananas should be avoided if you are allergic to ragweed.
b) If you have a known allergy to grasses, it will help to avoid wheat and other grains in the spring when grains and grasses bloom.
c) Some women react adversely to certain foods during a particular phase of their menstrual cycle. In other words a variable allergic reaction may occur monthly, seasonally, or otherwise and has a layered cause. The reason for this variability is multiple stressors – also known as the "total load".

Examples of what specific food allergies can cause:

- Pork allergy can trigger allergic arthritis.
- Citrus allergy can cause genitourinary problems and urinary tract infections.
- Yeast and mold allergy can trigger skin rashes, asthma, bloating and gastritis. They can also lead to susceptibility to yeast infections in women.

- Egg allergy can trigger headaches, migraines, hives and skin rashes.
- Milk allergy can lead to recurrent ear infections, post nasal drip, sneezing, leg aches and stomach aches.
- Soy allergies can cause gas, bloating and intestinal cramping.
- Tomato and wheat allergies can trigger inflammatory bowel disease or Crohn's Disease.

Conditions That Allergies Can Cause

When allergies have been long-term or chronic, the body can react in ways that don't seem like allergy reactions. It's like a mask or disguise with a different face. The following conditions are examples of "other faces" of allergies or sensitivities.

"Leaky Gut" Syndrome

This is an odd term with a literal meaning. The gut or the small intestines actually begins to leak undigested protein molecules into the bloodstream. Due to food allergies, sensitivities, yeast or parasites, the lining of the intestinal wall wears away, and tears or lesions result. Large protein molecules then slip through the lining and enter the bloodstream, undigested. The immune system then attacks them as unknown or foreign invaders, thus causing malabsorption of nutrients, allergic reactions, digestive and bowel problems and fatigue.

This process may also create a morphine-like effect that can disturb speech and auditory processing, causing a child to zone out or withdraw from others.[16] Avoidance of allergic foods and healing the "gut" lining is of the utmost importance here. A deficit in how a child processes information may be nothing more than chronic allergies and intestinal damage. The good news is the lining can be repaired with nutritional support, such as probiotics, whey, and the amino acid, L-glutamine.

Brain Allergies

Another type of allergy not commonly discussed, is called a brain allergy. In his book, *Brain Allergies*, William H. Philpott, M.D. presents many discussions and studies on this topic. He and his predecessor, Theron Randolph, M.D., considered that 60-70 percent of symptoms diagnosed as psychosomatic were, in fact, undiagnosed maladaptive reactions to foods, chemicals and inhalants.[17] Exposure to these substances evoked symptoms ranging from mild central nervous system reactions, like dizziness, blurred vision, depression and anxiety, to gross psychotic symptoms such as catatonia, dissociation, paranoid delusions and visual and auditory hallucination. Brain allergies can also lead to unexplained fears, headaches, inability to read or write, hyperactivity, sleepiness and insomnia.[18]

I had a brilliant professor, James Croxton, who once said, "*Behind every twisted thought is a twisted molecule.*" This means that for all negative thoughts and emotions, there is a physiological link – and that can be spurred on by certain foods, such as wheat, corn, dairy and sugar.

Headaches and Allergies

Some of the foods listed below contain amines, which are chemicals found in proteins that often produce allergic reactions in the body. If these substances pass into the bloodstream, they may constrict blood vessels, causing pain and headaches.

Most any food, to which an individual is allergic, can cause a headache after it is ingested. Headaches may also be the result of your body's reaction to something inhaled -- perfumes, household cleaning products, auto pollution or industrial pollution. Or, you may have a bio-mechanical problem for which you might seek chiropractic care or cranial-sacral therapy.

Common foods contributing to headaches:

- Aged cheeses (cheddar, Swiss, bleu cheese, Roquefort, brie)
- Alcohol (especially wine and beer)
- Aspartame or NutraSweet
- Avocados (very ripe only)
- Bananas (very ripe only)
- Caffeine: coffee, tea, colas
- Chemical additives, colorings, preservatives (the words you can't pronounce)
- Chicken livers
- Chocolate
- Citrus fruits
- Dairy products (especially sour cream and yogurt)
- Dry-roasted peanuts
- Dry-roasted walnuts, cashews, pecans, pistachios and other tree nuts
- Eggs
- Fermented foods (vinegar, soy sauce)
- Instant and canned soups (contain MSG)
- Instant gravies and tenderizers
- Meat tenderizers

- Monosodium Glutamate (MSG) (ask your Chinese restaurant to leave it out!)
- Nitrates and Nitrites
- Onions
- Pickled foods (pickles, herring, beets, etc.)
- Processed luncheon meats, hot dogs, pepperoni, bologna
- Smoked meats (salami, ham, pastrami. corned beef, jerky)
- Strawberries
- Sugar
- Wheat products (breads, cakes, pastas, pastries)

Other headache-causing substances are amphetamines, barbiturates, recreational drugs, paint fumes, automobile exhaust, perfumes, and chemical or toxic inhalants.

Testing for Allergies

There is no 100 percent reliable test for food allergies. I speak to people daily, who are totally puzzled by results of test that they've taken. Usually, they remark that their allergy doctor did skin testing and they were negative for food allergies. Yet, they know they clearly react to certain foods. Other people try elimination diets and seem to have no clear cut results. Each of the following tests has its limitations or shortcomings and its benefits:

Elimination Diet or Food Re-Challenge - After a food is avoided for a time, at least 5-7 days, it is then reintroduced. There may be no initial response if the reaction happens to be cumulative or variable. The best that can be determined by a one time challenge is that the person must not have an immediate, fixed reaction to that food. A food challenge must be repeated several times over two days or so to rule out these other forms of food reaction.

Double-Blind Food Capsule Test - Although this test may work reasonably well for a fixed reaction on someone with a low threshold for that food, it is in general a very unreliable test for food reactivity. Studies have shown that this technique is successful in only a small percentage of cases.

Blood Test for Food Allergies - These are called RAST or radioallergosorbent tests. There are several medical laboratories that offer these blood tests for the identification of food allergies that measure IgE and IgG antibodies against foods. They are not 100% accurate, sometimes showing false positives and false negatives. Though sometimes considered controversial in the medical community, they can be valuable in identifying major food offenders....and are very useful, especially for children who won't sit still for skin testing.

Skin Testing - Various types of skin responses have been investigated and some are more valid than others:

The conventional skin "scratch" test - The doctor places a drop of the substance being tested on the patient's forearm or back and pricks the skin with a needle, allowing a tiny amount to enter the skin. If the patient is allergic to the substance, a wheal (mosquito bite-like bump) will form at the site within about 15 minutes. The skin "scratch" allergy testing does not work as well for food allergies as it does with environmental allergies, and it is also invasive and painful.

Electro Dermal Screening (EDS) is another type of skin testing, but it is non-invasive. It is a computerized test in which the practitioner checks acupuncture points on the skin of the hands or feet. This is a non-provocative type of screening, which does not present any risk of serious allergic reactions like the ones associated with traditional skin testing. It is the method of choice for many patients, especially children and severely allergic individuals, because it checks for a multitude of food ingredient and environmental substances not found in traditional allergy tests. It also allows for rapid screening of large numbers of allergens in a risk-free and painless way.

Treatment after receiving the electro dermal screening results may vary according to your practitioner. Specific food elimination for a period of time is helpful in order to give the immune system a rest from the bombardment of allergens it has had over the years. Most, if not all practitioners who use this screening method would advise this.

What differs in the treatment are the types of nutritional supplements and homeopathic preparations used. That is up to your practitioner. He or she has found what they, with their clinical experience, think works best. Go with that. Some people may see results in just a few weeks; for others, it may take a few months.

One type of treatment, called ***optimal dose neutralization*** is very successful. This is a sublingual (under the tongue) method using liquid drops which one takes according to the practitioner's recommendations. This type of treatment is not accompanied by the serious risk of allergic reactions associated with conventional allergy treatment.

Optimal dose neutralization may afford relatively rapid relief of symptoms and stabilization of the immune system. Effective management may require periodic re-assessment for the first few months of treatment. As the body changes, the type and potency of the neutralization drops must be changed in order for the body to adapt. Eventually, the allergy symptoms decrease or disappear.

5. Toxicity – Body Overload

Our bodies are built to handle toxins; they are all around us – in our food, air, and water. Proportionally, children eat more food, breathe more air, and drink more fluids than adults. This increases their exposure to environmental toxins.[19]

The problem is that when children are young, the usual protection systems that the body has designed are not mature yet.[20] These are the protective barriers of the intestines and the brain. In the intestines, the protective barrier is called the ***intestinal lining*** and in the brain, it is called the ***blood-brain barrier***. Both of these protective systems aid in keeping toxins away. The intestinal lining helps keep toxins from entering the bloodstream and the blood brain barrier helps keep toxins from entering the highly sensitive brain.

So, with increased exposure and reduced protection, children are more likely than adults to have cognitive and behavioral imbalances relating to toxins.[21,22] In other words, the toxins are more toxic, especially for young children.

There is no doubt that toxic overload in our environment has escalated in the last fifty years. Some people handle it better than others. However, now there are more allergies, immune susceptibilities and more inflammatory problems than ever. Our children are uncomfortable and we are "beside ourselves" because it affects how they think and how they behave.

These are the very children that may become slow detoxifiers, having a reduced ability to neutralize and eliminate toxins. They may be more reactive than children who can efficiently detoxify. Many autistic children for instance, have impaired detoxification systems, so chemicals, vaccines, allergens and drugs may not pass out of the body as quickly as they do with other children. Toxic build-up can cause:

- Inflammation, discomfort, pain
- Asthma, sinusitis, ear infections, respiratory problems, and congestion
- Skin problems, rashes, eczema, psoriasis
- Slower growth rate due to impaired uptake of nutrients
- Developmental delays
- Weight imbalances due to poor metabolism of carbohydrates, proteins or fats
- Cognitive, emotional, mental imbalances due to chemical reactions
- Interrupted sleep, nightmares, fear, sweats

- Energy imbalances due to poor metabolism of carbohydrates, proteins or fats
- Poor hormone conversion, causing hormonal imbalances
- Hyperactivity, fidgetiness, fear reactions, depression, inability to get along with peers or siblings

In order to enhance detoxification for children and teens, it is important to "open the channels". In other words, enhance the body's natural detoxification pathways – the lungs, liver, lymph system, bowels, kidneys and skin. This is vital in order to usher the toxins out of the body. Your practitioner can help direct you toward products that are appropriate for children and programs that are gentle, yet effective.

Facts About Toxic Chemicals

Total release of developmental chemicals and toxins in the U.S. is estimated at 24 billion pounds annually, according to a report by several organizations, including Physicians for Social Responsibility.[23,24] Wrap your mind around that. It is almost inconceivable.

These developmental toxins, such as benzenes, dioxins, toluene and PCB's, have the potential to affect the way a child's body and brain develop, especially in the womb. Now, the U.S. Census Bureau estimates that about 12 million American children under 18 -- one out of every six -- suffer from at least one developmental, behavioral or learning disability. These include mental retardation, birth defects, autism, developmental delays, ADD and ADHD.

The National Academy of Sciences estimated earlier this year that 3 percent of these developmental and neurological problems in children are caused by exposure to known toxic substances.[25] Most of these chemicals have not been adequately tested for their toxicity to humans, and far fewer for neuron-toxicity:

- Vaccinations – preservatives, toxic metals
- Prescription drugs, including antibiotics
- OTC drugs, baby aspirin, cough meds, Tylenol
- Alcohol or drugs in utero (fetal alcohol or drug syndrome)
- Accumulated toxic metals: cadmium, aluminum, lead, mercury, antimony, arsenic
- Food preservatives, food colorings, additives
- Foods contaminated with chemical fertilizers, pesticides and sprays
- Glues, strong cleaning/degreasing agents, paint strippers, paint, varnishes, sealants, art materials, gasoline (likely to contain solvents)

- Toluene, released by the printing industry (nerve and developmental toxin)
- Fumes, vapors, dusts, strong odors (solvents, metals) - found in detergents, drier sheets and scented air fresheners, as seen in the study below.

NIH Reports Toxin in Air Fresheners

Longnecker, EL, MP, et al, "Volatile Organic Compounds and Pulmonary Function", *Environ Health* Perspect 114:1210–1214 (2006).

Exposure to 1,4-DCB (1,4-dichlorobenzene), a volatile organic compound related to the use of air fresheners, toilet bowl deodorants, and mothballs, at levels found in the U.S. general population, may result in reduced pulmonary function. This common exposure may have long-term adverse effects on respiratory health.

In Harm's Way

The revealing paper, "In Harm's Way: Toxic Threats to Child Development" lays out compelling, scientifically-documented arguments about the steps we as a society can take to increase our understanding of nerve and brain toxicity of chemical agents in our environment. It also recommends adopting public health policies that limit the exposure of fetuses and children to environmental chemicals.[26]

Recommendations are:

- Expectant mothers should avoid eating tuna.
- Children should avoid eating foods high in animal fat: fast food, ice cream, cheese, whole milk, fatty meats and/or fish. These may contain PCB's or dioxin that accumulate in the fat tissues of our bodies.
- Children should avoid crawling on floors and carpets with chemical cleaners.
- Children should avoid playing and rolling in pesticide-ridden grass.
- Avoid living near hazardous waste sites or places with hazardous emissions.
- Air out clothing from dry cleaners before wearing.
- Get houses tested for lead, if painted before 1978.
- Check your water sources (see section about water in *Chapter 3*).

No One Cause

Toxin upon toxin. We don't really know the effects of multiple offenders. Imagine this scenario:

1. A child has Fruit Loops for breakfast, with sugar, artificial colors and preservatives. He or she is allergic to the low-fat milk on the cereal, but the parents don't know this.
2. The child's sinuses get congested from the milk and the cereal and his mom gives them an over-the-counter, drug-store-bought nasal spray with chemical anti-histamines, decongestants, and artificial preservatives and sweeteners.
3. He or she then puts on sunscreen and jumps in a chlorinated pool.
4. After swimming a while, he or she begins to cough, gets out of the pool, towel dries with a towel that has been washed with scented detergent and dried with scented, softening drier sheets.
5. He or she then goes in the chemically air-freshened house and takes a commercial cough syrup with a stimulant ingredient, artificial sweeteners, artificial colors and preservatives.
6. Afterwards, the child has a Diet Coke with aspartame, followed by commercial corn chips, with food coloring, MSG, and preservatives.
7. But, have no fear. The child does remember to brush his or her teeth – however, it is with colorful, artificially-sweetened toothpaste that contains fluoride.

Whoa – within 30 minutes, this child ingested a minimum of 100 different chemicals! Separately, these items may seem innocuous, but we're talking about layer upon layer of chemicals that are potentially harmful to the brain and nervous system. This happens continually, throughout each day.

The good news is that you can work with your doctor or health practitioner to strengthen the blood-cleansing organs: bowels, kidneys, lungs, skin and lymph system and support the liver, your toxin-elimination factory. Homeopathic preparations and nutritional supplement programs can be individualized for your children to enhance cleansing and supporting the organ systems.

The Best Nutrient is Elimination

And if your doctor doesn't know how to advise you about a more natural approach, there is so much you can do on your own. The best nutrient is really elimination of as many of the chemicals and allergens that are in your family's life. Start one room at a time or one product at a time. Your health food store will be a great source for toxin-free products, but many grocery stores are now getting “up to speed” with natural options. Of course, you can get anything online.

What You Put on Your Skin You Eat

What our skin and our bodies come into contact with in today’s squeaky-clean living is overwhelming. In fact, it is toxic bombardment. There is a hygienic or cleansing product for every part of our body and for every surface and item in your home, office and car. Toxic chemicals abound. We breathe them, lather with them, brush with them and soak in them. We touch them constantly. Without a doubt, we absorb them.

Just what is it we’re absorbing? Synthetic fragrances, artificial colors, ‘age-accelerating’ toxic chemicals and preservatives such as propylene glycol, sodium lauryl sulfate, toluene, mineral oil, parabens, imidazolidinyl and diazolidinyl urea and triethanolamine (TEA). These chemicals are known to cause a wide variety of symptoms including eye problems, allergies, skin irritations, headaches, liver, kidney and nervous system damage. And the accumulation just adds to our overall toxic load.

Due to public demand, an entire industry has been built on developing natural cleaning products --everything from non-toxic bathroom cleaners to environmentally friendly dish soaps. Seventh Generation, Planet, and Earth Friendly Products are examples of companies that have put a lot of effort and thought into their great products. But there are also tried and true natural ways to clean, if you want to save money or want to be creative. Here are some things to try:

- **Baking soda**: An all-purpose cleaner; effective on glass coffee pots and glassware; removes red-wine stains from carpeting. A paste (made with water) can shine stainless steel and silver and remove tea stains from cups and saucers. Add Castile or vegetable-based liquid soap and a drop of essential oil (tea tree or lavender) to clean sinks, countertops, toilets and tubs.
- **Coarse salt**: Cleans copper pans and scours cookware. Sprinkle salt on fresh spills in the oven, and then wipe off. Sprinkle salt on rust stains and squeeze a lime or lemon over them, let sit for several hours and wipe off.
- **Grapefruit-seed extract**: Add to water in a spray bottle for an odorless way to kill mold and mildew.
- **Lemon juice**: Use as a bleaching agent on clothing and to remove grease from your stove and countertops. Add 2 tablespoons of lemon juice to 10 drops of real lemon oil plus 3 drops of jojoba oil to clean and polish wood furniture.

- **Olive oil:** Use to lubricate and polish wood furniture (three parts olive oil to one part vinegar; or two parts olive oil to one part lemon juice).
- **White vinegar:** Cleans linoleum floors and glass (from windows to shower doors) when mixed with water and a little liquid soap (Castile or vegetable). It cuts grease, removes stains and soap scum and cleans toilets. Pour down drains once a week for antibacterial cleansing. Add to water in a spray bottle to kill mold and mildew.
- **Tea tree oil**: Add to vinegar/water solutions for antibacterial properties. Use to kill mold and mildew, and on kitchen and bathroom surfaces. Add 50 drops to a bucket of water to clean countertops and tile floors.

Sunscreens

We would be remiss if we didn't comment on sunscreens. It is politically incorrect to advise against using sunscreen, but ah, what the heck. Don't use sunscreen. Unless you use a non-toxic version, commercial sunscreens are full of chemicals and they do absorb through the skin. They are worse than damage from the sun in many ways, and they block the UVB rays which are necessary for producing vitamin D3 in the skin. They also contain xenoestrogens, man made estrogen-like substances, as ingredients.

Instead:

- Use light colored clothing that reflects sun's rays.
- Try a natural sunscreen such as Aubrey's Green Tea Sunblock for Children SPF 25 from the health food store.
- Try All Terrain's Kids' Sport SPF 30 – PABA and paraben-free, complete UVA and UVB protection, from your health food store.

Insect Repellants

Bug repellants that contain DEET are very toxic. They can cause severe allergic reactions and lead to unnecessary toxic build-up in the body. Here are other options that you can buy from outdoor stores or your health food store:

- Kid's Herbal Armour by All Terrain – award-winning, DEET-free repellant
- Aubrey's Gone – safe bug repellant with powerful blend of herbal oils, no pesticides or petrochemicals
- Anti-Bug Balm by Badger with essential oils and DEET-free, for deep woods and swamp areas
- Swy Flotter by Kiss My Face – DEET-free, no artificial colors, fragrances, parabens

Homemade Bug Repellant

- 4 drops lavender
- 4 drops eucalyptus
- 4 drops tea tree oil
- 1 teaspoon witch hazel
- 4 teaspoons water

Remember, what you put on your skin you eat! Be scrutinizing with your choice of body care and household products, for yourself and your family.

6. Metabolic Imbalances

Metabolic imbalances involve multiple systems of the body. These imbalances result in the body's inability to burn fuel for energy. Food is our fuel and if you eat the wrong foods for you, or if you don't metabolize them well, your cells will not produce energy. The furnace will not turn on; calories will not burn efficiently; energy production will be impaired.

Metabolic Syndrome

An estimated one in ten 12-19-year-old adolescents in the United States has Metabolic Syndrome.[27] It is a condition that reflects the diet of our times – the focus on carbohydrates, sugar and fats. It is not a disease, but a collection of symptoms used to predict cardiovascular disease, growth, obesity and blood sugar disturbances.

A person with Metabolic Syndrome is defined as having an increased risk of cardiovascular disease and type 2 diabetes. Other conditions associated with it are high blood pressure, gallstones, asthma, sleep disturbances, insulin resistance, polycystic ovary syndrome and some forms of cancer. Underlying factors are inactivity, abdominal obesity and a high fat, high sugar diet.

Metabolic Syndrome, emerging mostly in adults in the last thirty years, is now considered a problem for many adolescents. It has doubled in the last decade, probably due to the 50 percent increase in adolescent obesity in the same time period.

Early Signs of Disease in Adolescents

Pediatric Ann. 2006 Dec; 35(12):898-902, 905-7.

"Metabolic Syndrome" may be present in as many as 30% of obese adolescents. It is manifested by the coexistence of central obesity (main body fat is centralized around the abdomen), blood lipid imbalances, hypertension and pre-diabetes.

New criteria have been generated for Metabolic Syndrome in adolescents, as seen in the February 2007 issue of the *Journal of the American College of Cardiology*. A person with metabolic syndrome must meet at least 3 of the following criteria, especially elevated waist circumference.[28]

- Increased waist circumference
- Higher than normal blood pressure
- Low HDL or good cholesterol
- High triglycerides
- Higher than normal fasting glucose

We advise a low glycemic diet for children and teens with Metabolic Syndrome. (See *Special Diets Chapter 11*.) Staying with good fats and cutting the bad fats is also important.

Sedentary children and teens are most at risk for developing this syndrome. Of equal importance is physical activity. Regular physical movement, sports or individual exercise programs are imperative for reversing Metabolic Syndrome and preventing diseases down the road. Reversal is possible. No one is doomed. It just requires logic, persistence, and good information to improve health.

Obesity: Growing Children, Growing Trend

Obesity has reached epidemic proportions among the population of children in North America in the last decade. From 2003 to 2004, about 17.1 percent of children and adolescents ages 2 to 19 in the United States, or 12.5 million kids, were considered overweight by the U.S. Centers for Disease Control and Prevention.

Overweight adolescents often become obese adults:

- Approximately 16% of children and adolescents ages 6-19 are overweight.[29]
- The prevalence of overweight among children aged 6-11 years has more than doubled in the past 20 years and among adolescents aged 12-19 has more than tripled.[30]
- Though the prevalence of overweight and obesity has increased in all segments of the U.S. population, it is particularly common in minority groups.[31]
- While America isn't alone in this trend, it does have the highest prevalence of obesity among developed nations.[32]
- Obesity is a condition in which a person's body weight is 20% above average for his or her age and frame size. Many health risks are not far behind:

- If your 5-year old child is overweight, he or she has a 20% chance of becoming obese as an adult.
- If your teenager is overweight, he or she has a 75% chance of becoming an obese adult!
- An estimated 60% of 5- to 10-year-old obese children already have one associated cardiovascular disease risk factor, and more than 20% have two or more risk factors.[33]
- Increased weight during middle childhood increases the risk of developing asthma by as much as 50%.[34]

Breakfast Matters for Weight Balance

Timlin MT et al. "Breakfast eating and weight change in a 5-year prospective analysis of adolescents: Project EAT (Eating Among Teens)." *Pediatrics* 2008 Mar; 121:e638.

In a 5-year study, investigators examined the association between breakfast eating patterns on BMI and weight changes in 2216 adolescents (55% girls, 63% white) at the mean age of 15 and again at 19.

Adolescents who ate breakfast daily had lower BMIs than those who never or intermittently ate breakfast. An estimated 25% of U.S. children regularly skip breakfast, the researchers said.

Conclusion: The results indicate that missing breakfast is associated with weight gain.

No One Cause

Many of the problems discussed in this chapter can lead to obesity: blood sugar imbalance, nutrient deficiencies and the list goes on. But, the basic cause of obesity in children is probably lack of exercise. Surely, the fact that physical education classes in the public school systems have decreased by a whopping 80% in just the past few years, is one reason. "Couch Potato Syndrome" and the excessive focus on computer use and TV-viewing are other logical reasons.

An enormous contributing factor to obesity in children is malnutrition, or under-eating of nutrient-rich food. We over-eat foods that are nutritionally empty and under-eat foods that are nutrient-rich. Obese and overweight children should eliminate empty calorie foods such as pizza and limit beverage intake. Most beverages, except water, contribute to excess calorie intake. Diet beverages don't work. Ridden with artificial sweeteners and colors, they are toxic to the nervous system and the brain. Isn't it ironic that so many people drink diet sodas and our society is fatter than ever?

Did Microwaves Kick-Start the Obesity Epidemic?

According to some experts, the answer is YES. Professor Jane Wardle at the University College, London, says that the rapid rise in obesity rates could be related to the widespread ownership of microwave ovens. Obesity rates started to rise soon after 1984, at about the same time as the microwave became a common household item.[35] Professor Tim Lang argued that the introduction of the supermarket was the cause. Meanwhile, Professor Ken Fox posited that the obesity epidemic can be traced back to 1945, when technology began to replace physical effort in work and leisure.

So, no, microwaves are not the sole source of the obesity problem, but they can be a detriment to one's health. Here's why. They can:

- Cause food to lose vital cancer-fighting nutrients like antioxidants and flavonoids.
- Satisfy the need for instant gratification, so they are used often for nutrient-deficient, ready-made meals.
- Release carcinogenic toxins from paper plates or plastic covers into your food.
- Change the chemical structure of your food, depleting enzymes and changing the molecular structure of fatty acids, with unknown consequences.

Corn Syrup

Another reason for the epidemic proportions of obesity is high fructose corn syrup, the #1 leading source of calories in the U.S. It is the most prevalent sweetener used today, especially in beverages: energy & sports drinks, fruit drinks, fruit juices and sodas. Sodas are being purchased from vending machines in the schools, by the liter or gallon for home, and by the Big Gulp on the run. When you add physical inactivity to the equation, the insulin receptors in the body become desensitized, causing a cascading that leads to weight gain. The following review exposes these issues:

"The 'skinny' on childhood obesity: how our western environment starves kids' brains." Lustig RH. Division of Endo, UCSF Center for Obesity Assessment, Study and Treatment, Pediatric Annals 35:12 , December 2006, 898-907

In this review, the author discusses the use of refined carbohydrates, such as high fructose corn syrup and how we store fat due to improper insulin use. This results in weight gain and a sense of starvation, which causes reduced energy and physical activity, and further promotes obesity. Dr. Lustig suggests:

-- Exercise by playing, walking, bike riding, playing sports (at least 30 minutes a day).
-- Stop buying sweets and soda.
-- Have your children help you prepare meals. Make a game of it. Ask them, "What vitamin does this carrot contain?" Plant the seeds to help them make better choices.
-- Limit TV time to help with the addiction of tuning out and being lazy.
-- Plan activities - a trip to the library, playground or park. Keep moving.

Also, high fructose corn syrup use can lead to Type-2 diabetes, hypertension and high triglycerides in the blood.[36] It can be a severe and sometimes hidden allergen for some children, to add another dimension to the mix.

Further research indicates that corn syrup and other processed foods are key reasons for the obesity epidemic because they promote hormonal imbalances that encourage children to overeat.[37]

Obesity, Insulin, and the "New Hormone": Leptin

"Childhood obesity: behavioral aberration or biochemical drive? Reinterpreting the First Law of Thermodynamics", Lustig, RH, MD, *Nature Clinical Practice Endocrinology & Metabolism* (2006) 2, 447-458.

Diseases that once were only seen in adults, like Type-2 diabetes, now are occurring in increasing numbers in children. Overweight kids often become overweight adults, which also puts them at greater risk of high blood pressure, heart disease and stroke. Children who are obese can be socially ostracized and teased, putting them at risk for depression and other psychiatric conditions.

Dr. Lustig says that it has long been known that the hormone insulin acts on the brain to encourage eating in two ways. First, it blocks the signals that travel from the body's fat stores to the brain by suppressing the effectiveness of the hormone, leptin, resulting in increased food intake and decreased activity. Second, insulin promotes the signal that seeks the reward of eating carried by the chemical dopamine, which makes a person want to eat to get the pleasurable dopamine "rush."

Changes in food processing during the past 30 years, the addition of sugar to many foods that once never included sugar and the removal of fiber, have created an environment in which our foods are essentially addictive.

All in all, though I don't recommend eating sugar, it is a better choice than eating products containing high fructose corn syrup.

Obesity, Self-Esteem, Self-Image

An emotional demise is associated with obesity. In fact, it is just as burdensome as the physical health consequences, as is seen in the following study.

> **"Fatso, Fatty, Blimp"**
> "The Relationship Between Relative Weight and School Attendance Among Elementary Schoolchildren", Geier, AB, Foster, GD, Womble, LG, McLaughlin, J, et al, *Obesity* 15:2157-2161 (2007)
>
> Overweight and obese children show a tendency to be absent from school more often than other children. This study suggests that the overweight children miss more days of school than normal weight or underweight children, in order to avoid being called names or bullied.[38]

Overweight children tend to have very poor self-images. Anorexia and bulimia (self-starvation and binge-eating followed by vomiting) are major problems among adolescent girls today. Eating habits and skewed self-images that lead to these problems are being formed in childhood, due to diet products, advertising and TV.

Early stages of several "adult diseases" are being observed in young obese people today. Cardiovascular disease, arthritis, cancer, high cholesterol, diabetes and metabolic syndrome are the more severe examples.

What is down the road for these kids? Where does it all lead? It's time to get a hold of ourselves and realize that the physical and emotional issues accompanying obesity are rooted in dietary and metabolic or hormonal problems. The next section may shed some light on the subject and give you food, not only for thought, but for taking action.

7. Hormone Imbalances

Hormones are powerful chemical messengers manufactured by the glands in the body that are all part of the endocrine gland system. This system is a very complex network that helps us balance stress and react to our environment.

How would you know if your child had a hormone imbalance? Generally, hormones are not tested in children. This is one of the most highly overlooked areas in conventional pediatric practices. What happened on your child's last check up: Height, weight and temperature measured? A listen to the lungs? A look in the ears and throat? What about testing for energy imbalances, metabolic problems and stress hormone levels? A simple saliva test helps to indicate if any of these areas out of balance. And if they are, your child will show some of the signs listed below.

Adrenal Hormones

From body size to energy output to yes, even the sound of your voice, hormones exert a powerful influence over all physical, intellectual and emotional behavior. Taking a look at the cortisol and DHEA adrenal hormone levels through saliva testing can be extremely revealing. Saliva collection for hormone testing is totally non-invasive and done right in your home. Salivary hormone testing is used for all ages – young children, teens and adults.

This is especially useful if a child has allergies, asthma, ADD, ADHD, autism, depression, or is aggressive or violent. High and low output of the adrenal hormones may indicate hypoglycemia as well as difficulty dealing with stress. Some parents remark that their children always seem to be in the state of "fight or flight", living on the edge. Below are other indicators of adrenal hormone imbalance:

Abnormal adrenal rhythm can influence:

- Bone, muscle and joint health
- Energy production
- Growth patterns
- Immune system health
- Skin regeneration
- Sleep quality
- Thyroid and metabolic function

Adrenal testing may be advised for individuals who suffer from:

- Alcohol intolerance
- Allergies & immune weakness
- Chronic stress and related health problems
- Depression and mood swings
- Fatigue, lack of vitality or endurance
- Growth problems
- Hypoglycemia
- Irritability and anxiety
- Low body temperature
- Low sex drive
- Migraine headaches
- Muscle and joint pain

- Poor memory or focus
- Sexual dysfunctions or precocious puberty
- Sleep disturbances
- Unexplained fear
- Weight control problems

Children, teens, PMS sufferers and high school athletes usually experience significant health changes due to stress and adrenal insufficiency. Many of the conditions associated with depression, anxiety, mood swings, focus and stress can be corrected with natural endocrine and nutrient creams, and/or nutritional therapies.

An innovative laboratory, Sabre Sciences in Carlsbad, California, custom-makes natural plant-based hormone and nutrient creams which are used topically. Absorbed through the skin into the bloodstream, these creams offer natural hormone precursors – building blocks that help to balance a variety of problems: energy levels, mood disorders, aggression, depression, insomnia, PMS, metabolic imbalances, growth problems and other associated conditions. I have seen exceptional results with this approach for children diagnosed with ADD, ADHD, autism, developmental delays, learning challenges and behavior problems.

Thyroid Hormones

The great ruler of metabolism - what a job the thyroid has! It affects energy, growth, and how we burn calories. If it is out of balance, it can accelerate its output of hormones. Over time, this can cause fatigue, weight problems, insomnia, dry hair and skin, cold hands and feet, lack of clarity and depression.

The thyroid may then slow down and under-produce its hormones. This is called hypothyroidism, low functioning of the thyroid gland (the gland of metabolism) causing sluggishness, fatigue, "foggy thinking", memory problems, weight gain and low body temperature. Hypothyroidism is sometimes associated with ADD. Thyroid hormone blood testing may reveal an imbalance. The most important thyroid test to get to determine this is the TSH or thyroid-stimulating hormone. If it is high, then the thyroid is under-producing its hormones.

Another test, easier to perform, is done using a basal thermometer first thing in the morning. Leave it in your mouth while you are still reclined and wait for it to beep. If the temperature is below 97.5, then it may indicate hypothyroidism. This is relative though. It is best to determine this with a knowledgeable health practitioner before jumping to conclusions. Many children with ADD and low thyroid levels improve thyroid function with a clean diet and appropriate nutritional supplementation. Eliminating food additives and dyes, especially red food dyes is vital, as they are toxic to the thyroid. Soy products also have a suppressive effect on the out-put of thyroid hormone.

Hyperthyroidism is characterized by an overactive thyroid gland, high blood pressure, accelerated heartbeat, hyperactivity, poor sleep habits and is sometimes associated with ADHD. The thyroid can be over-stimulated by high iodine intake through salt in fast foods as well as other sources. Getting the thyroid hormones tested through blood analysis is advised.

Grave's disease is a form of hyperthyroidism characterized by sweating, muscle weakness, tremors, fatigue and fast, irregular heart rate. It is often cause by exposure to toxins or poisons. Aspartame or NutraSweet is one of those toxins. In other words, Grave's disease can be the result too much aspartame in the diet.[39]

As far as treatment, there are different approaches for hyperthyroidism. For some children, medication for hyperthyroidism is prescribed. Depending on the severity of the condition, doctors might take the "wait and see" approach.

In other cases, the hyperthyroid condition may actually be thyroiditis, or inflammation of the thyroid gland. More often than not, the root cause is infection. A recent or current viral or bacterial infection can cause a temporary condition that your health care professional can treat. Natural anti-biotics or anti-virals can be implemented as well.

As a reminder, remember from the section on celiac disease in this chapter, that thyroiditis or high thyroid antibodies may indicate gluten sensitivity. With any hyperthyroid condition, it is wise to eliminate gluten-containing foods.

Last but not least, adrenal gland imbalance is always implied with thyroid imbalance. I usually suggest the salivary adrenal testing and treatment with adrenal balancing creams or supplements, in order to normalize the thyroid. This is imperative along with eliminating iodine-containing fast food. Remember that the glands and hormones work in a network, so assessing the network and balancing the glands that interconnect may solve the problem.

Reproductive Hormones

The reproductive hormones are estrogen, progesterone and testosterone. We all have ALL of them – boys, girls, men and women. They are manufactured by the sex organs, the testes in boys and men, and the ovaries in girls and women at varying levels, depending upon age. In this section, we'll examine several issues that affect the hormonal balance of our children and teens.

Premature or Precocious Puberty

Can you tell? The hormones are flying – certainly at earlier ages than I can remember. Science tells us that the age of puberty, the transition between childhood and adulthood, is becoming progressively younger for girls and boys.

Why Are Kids Entering Puberty Before They Enter School?
New York Times, October 17, 2006

This article revealed separate incidents in various countries where very young children had symptoms of early puberty: development of pubic hair and breast enlargement. Some children were found to have these symptoms from eating beef and poultry contaminated with estrogens and from other accidental drug exposure. Others reportedly displayed symptoms due to endocrine disruptors such as cosmetics, industrial pollutants and other environmental contaminants.

Puberty effects onset of menstruation (menarche), growth of breasts, genitals and pubic hair. Early puberty is defined in girls as under the age of 8 and in boys as under the age of 9. The following study shows premature puberty in girls today:

Early Breast and Pubic Hair Development in Girls-
Herman-Giddens, ME, et al, "Secondary sexual characteristics and menses in young girls seen in office practice: a study from the pediatric research in office settings network," April 1997, *Journal of Pediatrics*, Vol. 99(4):505-512.

Girls are developing breasts and/or pubic hair 6 months to a year sooner than science had previously determined. The age of menses has advanced by almost one-half year, especially in African American girls. The study suggests that early puberty and disruption of the hormonal system may be effected by the increasing use of certain plastics and insecticides that degrade into substances which have estrogen-related physiological effects on living things.

The same holds true for boys:

Secondary Sexual Characteristics in Boys at Younger Ages
"Estimates from the National Health and Nutrition Examination Survey III, 1988-1994", Herman-Giddens, ME, Wang L, Koch, G, *Arch Pediatr Adolesc Med.* 2001; 155:1022-1028.

A study of over 2,000 boys, ages 8-19, indicates that the average age of onset of genital and pubic hair growth were younger than in past studies. Additional studies are required to explore public health implications.

The childhoods of U.S. girls have been significantly shortened. Girls get their first periods, on average, a few months earlier than girls 40 years ago, but they get their breasts one to two years earlier.

Among U.S. white girls, the average age of onset of the period has declined over the past four decades and now stands at 12.6 years. Among U.S black girls, average age is 12.1 years and the ongoing rate of decline is swifter. This is also true among Mexican American girls. Similarly, the average age of breast and pubic hair growth has continued to fall among all groups and with significant ethnic/racial differences. About half of all U.S. girls show signs of breast development by their 10th birthday, with 14 percent attaining breast buds between their eighth and ninth birthdays.[40]

There is no single cause of early puberty. It may result from a variety of stressors --- some psychosocial, some nutritional, some chemical. They interact in young girls' bodies in ways that can accelerate maturation. Factors that may contribute to early puberty[41]:

- environmental exposures to endocrine-disrupting chemicals, such as pesticides, fungicides, plastics, beauty and personal care products, lawn care products and dental sealants
- low birth weight
- obesity and high calorie diets
- overweight
- premature birth
- reduced breastfeeding (Breast milk contains melatonin, which inhibits puberty.)
- smoking or breathing passive smoke
- use of infant soy formulas, containing estrogens (see next study below)

Estrogens in Infant Soy Formula

Irvine, C. et al., "The Potential Adverse Effects of Soybean Phytoestrogens in Infant Feeding", *New Zealand Medical Journal,* May 24, 1995, p. 318.

It is estimated that an infant exclusively fed soy formula receives the estrogenic equivalent (based on body weight) to at least 5 birth control pills per day.

Other factors currently under investigation include:

- physical inactivity
- psychosocial stressors, including father absence and family dysfunction[42]
- television viewing and media use

Facts about the risks and effects of early puberty:

- Established risk factor for breast cancer. As age of the onset of the first period decreases, overall risk of breast cancer increases.[43]
- Early drug use, cigarette smoking and alcohol use.[44]
- Early sexual intercourse and risk of teenage pregnancy.[45]
- Tendency to experience anxiety, depression and low self-esteem.[46]
- Tendency to develop eating disorders.[47]
- Potential of developing polycystic ovary syndrome.[48]

Another effect of early puberty is the declining ratio of boys to girls in live births and the increase in birth defects among boys, especially in areas with a high usage of hormone-disrupting pesticides, herbicides and fungicides.

Contraceptive Hormones

More and more girls are using contraceptive hormones at young ages. These may take the form of a pill or patch. The most common is the birth control pill, which comes in many varieties and hormonal combinations. They contain artificial female hormones, estrogens and progestins. Understand that these prescription hormones begin to control the body. Now, obviously, this is the point. Contraceptive hormones do their job, which is to prevent ovulation; they also thicken the lining of the cervix, preparing a hostile environment for sperm. The result is prevention of fertilization. Parents and doctors advocate use of contraceptive hormones to prevent unwanted pregnancies and to eliminate problems associated with the menstrual cycle.

Seemingly superficial side effects which many people overlook are weight gain, water retention, acne and mood swings. These side effects represent deeper issues which result from hormonal imbalance and toxicity caused by the contraceptives. Worst of all is estrogen dominance which can cause weight gain, infertility and reproductive cancers, such as breast cancer. These are not superficial problems. Since hormone replacement for birth control has increased since the 1980's, so have infertility and reproductive cancers. There is a distinct relationship here.

Recent research has also linked oral contraceptives with heart disease. They have been found to cause cardiac plaque in the femoral and carotid arteries.

Oral Contraceptives Linked to Increased Carotid Plaque

Rietzschel E, et al "Anti-conceptive Drug Use and Increased Carotid and Femoral Plaque Prevalence", American Heart Association Meeting, Orlando, Fla., Nov 6, 2007; Abstract 3614.

The use of a combination oral estrogen-progestin contraceptive by otherwise healthy young women increases the prevalence of carotid and femoral artery plaques by 20% to 30% for every 10 years of use.
Use of the birth control pill also increased blood pressure between 4 - 9 mmHg, and there was reduced HDL (good) cholesterol and increased LDL (bad) cholesterol.

Personal and societal problems caused by unwanted pregnancy are real. This is why many of today's young women are using contraceptives. Unfortunately, most doctors don't know or don't tell their patients or their parents about the potentially devastating threats to their health. If it was your daughter, would you want to know? Would you want to be able to make an informed decision?

Polycystic Ovary Syndrome

PCOS or Polycystic Ovary Syndrome, a hormone imbalance among young girls and adults, is increasing day by day. PCOS or multiple cysts on the ovaries, is spurred on by high insulin levels causing insulin resistance, thereby stimulating an over-production of estrogen and/or testosterone. This condition comprises a set of symptoms that may include an inability to ovulate, growth of excess body hair, loss of hair on the head and weight gain, especially around the waist.

Lowering or normalizing insulin levels is vital for hormonal balance and elimination of PCOS. Reducing simple carbohydrates such as high-glycemic and refined foods is an important strategy for balancing insulin resistance, estrogen and androgen dominance. Using natural progesterone (which is usually deficient) may be important in order to put an end to ovarian cysts, fibroids, endometriosis, PMS, hot flashes, weight gain and depression. Ask your health care practitioner to test for hormonal levels and take it from there.

Obesity More than Doubles Testosterone in Pubertal Girls

"Obesity and Sex Steroid Changes across Puberty: Evidence for Marked Hyperandrogenemia in Pre- and Early Pubertal Obese Girls", McCartney, CR, et al, *Journal of Clinical Endocrinology and Metabolism*, 2007, Vol. 92, No. 2 430-436.

Girls who are obese at puberty have higher blood markers for testosterone and insulin, compared with normal-weight girls. This predisposes them to higher rates of polycystic ovarian syndrome, excess hair growth and diabetes. Resulting menstrual irregularities may also lead to infertility.

Kids and Steroid Drugs

Steroid drugs are hormones. About 2.7% of teenage boys and 5.3% of teenage girls have used steroid drugs.[49,50] Teenagers look up to pro athletes and movie stars and with this emulation can come a desire to look leaner, more muscular, lose weight and improve strength and endurance. Kids with eating disorders are often attracted to steroid use as well.

Steroid drugs in the form of injectables, creams, patches and tablets are easy to come by on the streets from drug dealers and from friends. They are even romanticized to some extent. There is a fearlessness that kids have today, because so many activities are so palpable due to the various forms of media.

But steroid abuse disrupts the normal production of hormones in the body, causing changes – some more reversible than others. Changes that can be reversed include reduced sperm production and shrinking of the testicles (testicular atrophy). Breast development or gynecomastia may be difficult to reverse. Male-pattern baldness that is steroid-induced may be very difficult to reverse. In one study of male bodybuilders, more than half had testicular atrophy and/or gynecomastia.

In the female body, anabolic steroids cause masculinization. Breast size and body fat decrease, the skin becomes coarse and acne develops, the clitoris enlarges, and the voice deepens. Women may experience excessive growth of body hair but lose scalp hair. With continued administration of steroids, some of these effects become much more difficult to reverse. (See *Chapter 12*.)

8. Neurotransmitter Imbalances

Millions of children, yes, millions are being prescribed anti-depressants, stimulants, anti-anxiety drugs and sleep medications for bi-polar disorder, ADHD, anxiety, violent behavior, depression and insomnia. When psychiatrists are interviewed about the use of multiple prescriptions in children as young as one year of age, they shrug their shoulders. They don't know what else to do. Families are distraught and in pain about the behavior and emotional imbalance in their children, and the doctors are just trying to help. Yet these drugs are being used without enough science to back up their efficacy or safety. And children are dying. Can't anyone think outside their box?

There is a whole world of answers out there, like the ones we are revealing in this chapter. The chemistry of the brain is indeed very complex, but can be altered --- obviously, for the positive. It can be balanced. **The brain chemicals are simply made of nutrients**. But the medical and psychiatric specialists don't know this, or don't use this logic. They haven't been educated about how to nutritionally feed the brain, even though there are many peer-reviewed studies about nutritional deficiencies leading to emotional and behavioral imbalances.

One such study in the *Journal of Child and Adolescent Psychopharmacology* found that mood disorders can be balanced with biologically active vitamins and minerals.[51] If you have a child who is on psychiatric medications, then seek a health professional who has access to neurotransmitter testing and knowledge about nutritional brain fortification.

Neurotransmitters or brain chemicals are manufactured by nerve cells in the brain and, believe it or not, even in the intestines (as we've seen in the *Chapter 3 about Digestion*). These brain chemicals communicate with or talk to each other, controlling emotions, moods, behavior, sleep, energy, movement and physical ability to experience pleasure, discomfort and pain.

Severe repercussions occur when the brain and the nervous system are penetrated by chemicals in our food and environment, vaccinations and drugs. They can cause deficits in the central nervous system and associated cranial nerves, effecting the overall functioning of the body. Our nervous system is connected to all our organs and glands. The resulting feedback then affects our neurotransmitters, which control behavior, emotions and cognitive function. Even the growth process can be thrown into turmoil.

Analysis through the urine can now provide precise information about neurotransmitter deficiencies or overloads. Brain chemistry is affected by stress, diet and the environment. It is individual, thus requiring individual solutions.

Neurotransmitter testing measures the brain chemicals associated with:

- ADD, ADHD
- Anxiety and panic attacks
- Autism
- Behavioral problems
- Depression
- Developmental Delays
- Fatigue
- Fibromyalgia
- Growth problems
- Inability to handle stress
- Insomnia
- Living in "fight or flight"
- Mood swings
- Obesity

- OCD (Obsessive Compulsive Disorder)
- Sensory Processing Disorder (taste, touch, hearing, smell)
- Unexplained fears

Testing helps to determine exactly which neurotransmitter levels are out of balance and which therapies are needed for an individualized treatment plan. Neurotransmitters are manufactured in the body from nutrients, such as amino acids, which can help balance the brain chemistry.

THE NEUROTRANSMITTERS: What They Do

The neurotransmitter names recognized by the public are serotonin, dopamine, GABA and epinephrine or adrenalin. There are more, as you'll see in the list below, of the main neurotransmitters and their functions:

Serotonin

Serotonin is the most widely studied neurotransmitter -- perhaps because it plays such a significant role in sleep, anxiety and depression. It is a precursor to melatonin, the sleep hormone. It is also your body's natural anti-depressant and that is why SSRI or serotonin reuptake inhibitor drugs are used to relieve depression. They help the body utilize serotonin better.

Some of these drugs are Prozac, Paxil, Celexa, Lexapro and Zoloft. When a drug ceases to "work", the dosage must be increased or another drug option must be taken. This is because they really don't "cure" the problem, they just apply a band-aid.

Since an estimated 8-9 percent of adolescents in the U.S. suffer from depression, examining the serotonin levels through neurotransmitter testing or other assessments is imperative. If your doctor doesn't do this screening, find one who does. Remember that girls are twice as likely as boys to develop depression during adolescence. If untreated, it can lead to academic failure, social isolation, promiscuity, drug and alcohol use and suicide.[52]

The good news is that certain amino acid supplements can help increase the body's supply of serotonin. Serotonin is a synthesized from the amino acid L-tryptophan, and the supplement, 5-HTP is its precursor. So, it can be effective for relieving anxiety, depression, sleep disorders and increased appetite. It has also been shown to be effective for a wide variety of conditions associated with binge eating and obesity, chronic headaches, excessive blood clotting and chronic pain.

These amino acid supplements are available from your health food store or from your health practitioner, but it is best to test first in order to know where to begin. Tryptophan-containing foods are: mushrooms, spinach, milk, turkey, lamb, halibut, snapper, salmon and scallops. Also iron-deficiency anemia can lead to serotonin deficiency because iron is necessary for its production.

Dopamine

ADHD, lack of motivation and depression are linked to low dopamine levels Schizophrenia and anxiety disorders have been linked to excess levels.

Certain drugs for ADHD, such as Ritalin increase the output of dopamine in the brain, causing kids to be more interested in tasks presented to them, have better focus, alertness, and more compliance.[53]

Dopamine is also involved in sexual stimulation. High dopamine levels can cause someone to act "over-sexed" and low dopamine levels can cause low sex drive. On the other hand, low dopamine levels may lead a person to take more risks, in an effort to be stimulated. In other words, it may take more to stimulate them. This can lead to addictive behavior in several areas – searching for "the high".

Vegetarians, especially vegans may also be deficient in dopamine because of their low intake of protein. Foods that enhance its production are wild game meat, turkey, fish, beef, eggs, cheese and oats.

GABA

GABA or gamma amino benzoic acid is a predominant inhibitory or relaxing neurotransmitter. With imbalances, a person may have anxiety, depression or insomnia. Foods that may enhance GABA production are rice, oats, barley, halibut, nuts, beans and spinach.

Epinephrine or Adrenalin

This neurotransmitter also functions as a stress hormone. If levels are low, a child may have low energy, or an inability to handle stress. In other words, stress may be more stressful for that person. They may have more fears, nightmares and fatigue. Low epinephrine levels may also contribute to poor memory or information retrieval.[54] Excess caffeine and sugar can cause epinephrine imbalance.

Norepinephrine or Noradrenalin

Norepinephrine is synthesized by the amino acids L-phenylalanine and L-tyrosine, along with vitamins B6, C and niacin. It controls the release of the hormones that regulate sex and metabolism. Norepinephrine is also involved in sleep patterns, learning and memory. If norepinephrine levels are high, a person may have high blood pressure, anxiety or hyperactivity. In adults, high norepinephrine may lead to erectile dysfunction.

PEA or Beta Phenylethylamine

PEA is involved in focus and concentration problems and is often low in individuals with ADD and ADHD.[55]

Acetylcholine

This neurotransmitter is synthesized in the body by choline, lecithin, DMAE and vitamin co-factors such as C and B6. Foods that can enhance its production are eggs (yolk), cream and nuts. It is important in the role of behavior and memory; low levels of acetylcholine may result in forgetfulness. It is the most abundant neurotransmitter in the body and controls muscular activity. It is often very high in people with Parkinson's disease.

Taurine

Taurine is a relaxing neurotransmitter. It helps calm the nervous system, so it is used for hyperactivity, fidgetiness, anxiety and insomnia. Taurine is also an amino acid, so it is readily available in nutritional supplements.

It is currently being studied for use in bi-polar disorder by Dr. Andrew L. Stoll, associate professor of Psychiatry at Harvard. Dr. Stoll has explored amino acid supplements, specifically taurine, but the results have not yet been published. Dr. Stoll said, "It works really well for bipolar disorder." [56]

Glutamine

This amino acid serves as the precursor to glutamate and GABA. Optimal glutamine levels are important for the production of these two important neurotransmitters, as well as for intestinal function and repair. Significantly elevated glutamine levels may indicate imbalance in the nervous system. High levels may occur with dietary supplementation of glutamine.

Histamine

This is an excitatory neurotransmitter that can affect epinephrine and norepinephrine. High levels are associated with restlessness, stress, serotonin depletion, cigarette use and active allergies or inflammation. Low levels are associated with fatigue, low mood and antihistamine use.

Summary

In summary, many children have learning disabilities, emotional problems and/or behavioral disorders because of neurotransmitter imbalances. They may likely suffer from low self esteem or under-achievement in school. They may also develop social or relationship problems. When they get older, they may be prone to substance abuse and develop anxiety or other psychiatric disorders.[57]

As a result of testing, your health practitioner may suggest dietary changes, such as a balanced protein and carbohydrate diet. He or she may also suggest certain nutritional supplements that enhance digestion and absorption, improve circulation to the brain, and support the manufacture of the specific brain chemicals.

---

1. *American Diabetes Association, Statistics 2005, http://www.diabetes.org/diabetes-statistics/prevalence.jsp*
2. *Diabetes Care 2000;23:1348-1352*
3. *US News.com - from U.S News: A World Report, "Diabetic Kids Face Adult Burdens", Marcus, Mary Brophy, June 25, 2001.*
4. *Venkat, Narayan KM, Boyle JP, Thompson TJ, Sorensen SW, Williamson DF, "Lifetime Risk for Diabetes Mellitus in the US, Journal of American Medical Assoc, 2003; 290(14):1884-1890.*
5. *"Chronic Conditions; A Challenge for the 21st Century". National Academy on an Aging Society, 2000.*
6. *Summary of Health Statistics of US Children: National Health Interview Survey, 2002, www.cdc.gov/nchs*
7. *IBID*
8. *CDC. Fast Stats A-Z, Vital and Health Statistics, Series 10, no. 13. 1999. Web: http://www.cdc.gov/nchs/fastats/allergies.htm*
9. *Foresi A. A comparison of the clinical efficacy and safety of intranasal fluticasone propionate and antihistamines in the treatment of rhinitis. Allergy. 2000; 55:12-14.*
10. *Bousquet J, Van Cauwenberge P, Khaltaev N; Aria Workshop Group; World Health Organization. Allergic rhinitis and its impact on asthma. J Allergy Clin Immunol. 2001; 108(5 suppl):S147-S334.*
11. *Sibbald B, Rink E. Epidemiology of seasonal and perennial rhinitis: clinical presentation and medical history. Thorax. 1991; 46:895-901.*
12. *Celiac Disease Foundation, Studio City, CA, 818-990-2354, www.celiac.org*
13. *"Prevalence of Celiac Disease in At-Risk and Not-At-Risk Groups in the United States" Alessio Fasano, MD; Irene Berti, MD; Tania Gerarduzzi, MD; Tarcisio Not, MD; Richard B. Colletti, MD; Archives of Internal Medicine, February 10, 2003;163:286-292*
14. *Bhadada, S. Bhansali, A., Kochhar, R., Shankar, A., Menon, A., Sinha, S., Dutta, PP., and Nain, C, Does every short stature child need screening for celiac disease? Gastroenterology [Online Early Articles]. doi:10.1111/j.1440-1746.2007.05261.*
15. *Guliter, Sefa et al., "Prevalence of celiac disease in patients with autoimmune thyroiditis in a Turkish population", World Journal of Gastroenterology, 2007; 13 (10)*
16. *Mast, C, "The Nutrition Link", Delicious Living Magazine, May 2008, p. 32*
17. *IBID*

18. *Philpott, William H, M.D. and Kalita, Dwight K, Ph.D, Brain Allergies: The Psychonutrient Connection, Keats Publishing, Inc, 1980, pp. 16-17.*
19. *Needleman, H.* and *Landrigan, P. Raising Children Toxic Free, Avon Books, 1994*
20. *Blaylock, R. Excitotoxins: The Taste that Kills, Health Press, 1994. pgs. 18-19.*
21. *Needleman, H. and Landrigan, P, Raising Children Toxic Free, Avon Books, 1994.*
22. *Bruno, Jeffrey, Ph.D., Edible Microalgae: A Review of the Health Research, Center for Nutritional Psychology Press, Pacifica, CA, 2001.*
23. *In Harm's Way: Toxic Threats to Child Development, Greater Boston Physicians for Social Responsibility, May 2000 Report.*
24. *www.ourstolenfuture.org*
25. *"They're Poisoning Our Kids", Wired News: Environmental News Service, Sept 8, 2000. (http://www.wired.com/news/print)*
26. *T. Schettler, J. Stern, F. Reich, M. Valenti, and D. Wallinga. "In Harm's Way: Toxic Threats to Child Development", Greater Boston Physicians for Social Responsibility (GBPSR). 139 pp. 2000. http://psr.igc.org/ihw-project.htm*
27. *Park YW, et al. "The metabolic syndrome prevalence and associated risk factor findings in the US population from the Third National Health and Nutrition Examination Survey, 1988-1994. Arch Intern Med 2003; 163:427-36.*
28. *"New Criteria for Diagnosing Metabolic Syndrome in Teens", Journal of American College of Cardiology, February 2007; 49:891-898.*
29. *Hedley AA, Ogden CL, Johnson CL, Carroll MD. Curtin LR, Flegal KM, "Prevalence of Overweight and Obesity Among US Children", document from U.S. Department of Health and Human Services, Centers for Disease Control and Prevention, 2005*
30. *IBID*
31. *IBID*
32. *Ogden CL, Carroll MD, Curtin LR, McDowell MA, Tabak CJ, Flegal KM. Prevalence of overweight and obesity in the United States, 1999—2004, Journal of American Medical Association 2006;295:1549--55.*
33. *"The Increase of Childhood Chronic Conditions in the US", James M. Perrin, MD; Sheila R. Bloom, MS; Steven L. Gortmaker, PhD, Journal of American Medical Association, 2007;297:2755-2759.*
34. *Flaherman V, Rutherford GW. A meta-analysis of the effect of high weight on asthma. Arch Dis Child. 2006 Apr; 91(4):334-9.*
35. *Wardle, J (Professor in the Department of Epidemiology and Public Health at University College London, UK), excerpted from a debate at Cheltenham Science Festival, BBC News, June 6, 2007.*
36. *Hallfrisch, H, et al., The Effects of Fructose on Blood Lipid Levels, American Journal of Clinical Nutrition, 37: 5, 1983, 740-748.*
37. *Lustig, RH, MD, University of California at San Francisco, Review of Obesity Research, 8-11-06, Nature Clinical Practice Endocrinology & Metabolism*
38. *"The Relationship Between Relative Weight and School Attendance Among Elementary Schoolchildren", Geier, AB, Foster, GD, Womble, LG, McLaughlin, J, et al, Obesity 15:2157-2161 (2007)*

39. *Dr. Janet Starr Hull, Sweet Poison: How The World's Most Popular Artificial Sweetener Is Killing Us, New Horizon Press, ISBN; 0-88282-164-4.*
40. *FOOTNOTE: "The Falling Age of Puberty in U.S. Girls", Steingraber S, PhD, Breast Cancer Fund Report, 2007*
41. *IBID*
42. *IBID*
43. *IBID*
44. *IBID*
45. *IBID*
46. *IBID*
47. *IBID*
48. *IBID*
49. *"Monitoring the Future: National Results on Adolescent Drug Use, Overview of Key Findings", Johnston, LD, PhD, et al, 2006, p. 43 U.S. Dept. of Health and Human Services, National Institutes of Health*
50. *"Cross-sectional Study of Female Students Reporting Anabolic Steroid Use", Elliot, DL, MD; Cheong, J, PhD; Moe, EL, PhD, MPH; Goldberg, L, MD, Arch Pediatr Adolesc Med. June 2007;161:572-577*
51. *"Treatment of mood lability and explosive rage with minerals and vitamins: two case studies in children.", Kaplan BJ, Crawford SG, Gardner B, Farrelly G, Journal of Child Adolesc Psychopharmacol, 2002 Fall;12(3):205-19.*
52. *"Active Kids Less Prone to Depression", Motl, R, Psychosomatic Medicine, May-June 2004; vol 66: pp 336-342.*
53. *"PET, SPECT Studies Find More Evidence of Dopamine's Role in ADHD", Schuster, L, Medscape Medical News, June 24, 2003, based on Society of Nuclear Medicine 50th Annual Meeting: Abstracts 117, presented June 22, 2003; abstracts 216 and 1544, presented June 23, 2003.*
54. *Hanna, G.L., Ornitz, E.M, and Hanharan, M, "Urinary epinephrine excretion during intelligence testing in Attention-Deficit Disorder and normal boys". Biological Psychiatry, Sept 15, 1996, 40(6); 553-555.*
55. *Baker GB, Bornstein RA, Rouget AC, Ashton SE, van Muyden JC, Coutts RT. Phenylethylaminergic mechanisms in Attention-Deficit Disorder. Biological Psychiatry, 1991 Jan 1;29(1):15-22*
56. *"Managing Bi-Polar Disorder", Hara Estroff Marano, Psychology Today, 1 Nov 2003, Article ID: 1322*
57. *"Evaluating Prescription Drugs used to Treat ADHD, Comparing Effectiveness: Safety and Price", (2005) Consumer Reports Best Buy Drugs, 1-24.*

~ ~ ~

PART THREE - THE SOLUTIONS: Reversing the Trend

Chapter Nine

HEALTHY SUBSTITUTES MADE EASY: An Exciting New World

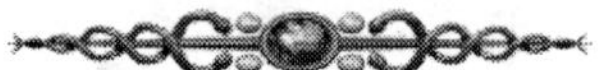

Why use food substitutions? Eliminate allergies, balance blood sugar, ingest more nutrient-rich food and improve focus and behavior. These are but a few great reasons to find substitute foods for what your family has been eating. The natural food industry has finally learned how to make these replacements taste good and some of them tasted good to begin with. It is an exciting world of food out there, with our many options!

Dairy and Dairy-Free Foods

Just taste the difference and you'll always want organic dairy products. Milk, cheese, butter, yogurt, sour cream and ice cream -- the organic dairy industry is skyrocketing in the U.S., Canada and Great Britain. Certainly anyone who is eating dairy products should be buying the organic ones – from companies such as Horizon Organics, Strauss Creamery, Clover and Organic Valley. Many grocery stores carry these products because consumer demand is high – and for very good reasons. The health benefits far outweigh non-organic dairy products and the toxic effects are far less.

Organic dairy products begin with organic farms. The food is produced without dangerous pesticides or chemicals; it is not irradiated, and genetically-modified organisms (GMO's) are not utilized. The cows are fed an organic, vegetarian diet. They are not given growth hormones or antibiotics. This issue is extremely significant for children. Children consume far more produce per pound of body weight than do adults. Evidence is increasing concerning the significant exponential toxicity of pesticides with children, because of their rapidly developing nervous systems.

Although some individuals benefit from organic cow's milk or dairy products, others do not. Dairy allergies, sensitivities and lactose intolerance are rampant. If you or your children are allergic or sensitive to cow's milk or dairy products, chose from the many non-dairy food substitutes for milk, cheese, butter, yogurt, sour cream and ice cream. Individuals with lactose intolerance and casein allergies can benefit equally from these alternative products. Casein is a phosphor-protein in milk that has a molecular structure extremely similar to that of gluten in some grains. Casein and gluten are equally troublesome to many individuals. They leak into the gut, undigested, and wreak havoc in the digestive and immune systems. Children and adults diagnosed with ADHD, autism, chronic fatigue syndrome, developmental delays, asthma and allergies are the most susceptible.

The number of children and adults with allergies and sensitivities to milk and dairy products is staggering. Some may not even realize they have an allergy or sensitivity. Common symptoms are ear infections, sinus problems, constant runny nose or clearing of the throat, asthma, eczema, skin rashes, diarrhea, constipation, gas, stomach aches, hyperactivity, depression, and many behavioral and emotional imbalances.

Milk Substitutes

Please keep in mind that ingredients change, so check any product before using. Look for dairy-free or casein-free on the label.

- Almond milk (vanilla, not original, chocolate and unsweetened)
- Amasake rice drink (Grainaissance)
- Better Than Milk - by Sovex Natural Foods – rice or soy dry mixes
- Blue Diamond Growers – Almond Breeze from almonds and tapioca starch
- Coconut milk – brands: So Delicious, Thai Kitchen, Wilderness Family Naturals (coconut water and milk, coconut cream, coconut milk powder)
- EdenBlend Milk – blend of organic soybeans and brown rice amasake milk
- Ener-G NutQuik powder – dry milk replacement from ground almonds
- Ener-G SoyQuik powder
- Hain Rice Supreme Drink
- Hazelnut Milk – Pacific brand
- Hemp Milk – derived from hemp seeds and made by Living Harvest
- MimicCreme – Nut-based, non dairy, non soy, vegan cream substitute
- Oat milk – Pacific brand
- Pacific brand – rice, oat and almond milks
- Power Dream Soy Energy Drinks - all varieties
- Rice milk - Rice Dream (Imagine Foods) – many flavors and brands, Pacific, Westbrae, White Wave
- Sovex Rice Moo
- Solait – instant soy beverage from Devansoy Farms
- So Nice - 100% organic, non-genetically modified soybeans are used
- Soy Dream Non-Dairy Beverages - all varieties
- SoyGood (soy based alternative)

- Vance's DariFree (see DariFree) – "milk" powder from maltodextrin, derived from potatoes - free of gluten, casein, soy, rice and MSG
- Vitasoy soy milk – many flavors and varieties
- Westbrae Rice Non-Dairy Drink
- Westsoy Soy Milk (nonfat, unsweetened)
- White Wave – Silk Soy Milk

Protein powders can be whipped up with water or any type of milk to nutritionally potentize a drink. Whey protein powder, a creamy, dairy-derived protein, is often tolerated by those with a dairy allergy or sensitivity. Goat whey is an especially viable source of protein. There are many varieties of whey protein, so find one that is unsweetened. You can sweeten it yourself with stevia, FOS, or agave. Protein powders, especially those marketed to athletes, contain hidden, artificial sweeteners such as acesulfame-K and aspartame. Rice and hemp proteins are also dairy-free alternatives and can be purchased from your local health food store or from your health care practitioner.

About Goat Milk Products

Some people with dairy allergies can tolerate goat milk products. Some can't. As an alternative, goat milk contains only trace amounts of alpha S1 casein, the major protein in cow's milk to which people are allergic. Goat milk also resembles more closely human milk than cow's milk. It has a softer curd; therefore, the fat globules do not cluster and are more digestible.

The fat globules in goat milk are also smaller than those in cow's milk. Because it easier to digest, some people who are lactose intolerant can handle goat milk.

Goat milk also contains significantly different fatty acids than cow's milk. It is high in caprylic, capric, lauric, myristic and palmitiric acids, which can uniquely assist in lowering cholesterol and improving cardiovascular function.

The nutrient content of goat milk is also better than cow's milk. It contains 13% more calcium that cow's milk, 47% more vitamin A, 350% more niacin, 25% more vitamin B6 and 34% more potassium. It is also a better source of selenium and electrolytes.[1]

Other goat products include varieties of cheese, yogurt, butter, whey and ice cream.

Ice Cream

- Cuties - soy ice cream bars
- Double Rainbow Dairy-Free Sorbets

- FreeZees – derived from nut butter, several flavors
- Fruit-based ice pops – Whole Foods Market
- Fruit Pops - Cascadian Farms
- Fudge Bars - Sweet Nothings
- Ice Bean - soy ice cream bars and pints
- Lil' Dreamers - vanilla and chocolate
- Organic Soy Delicious - pints and quarts, various flavors
- Purely Decadent – coconut milk ice cream in various flavors
- Rice Dream - frozen bars, pints, many flavors
- Soy Dream Frozen Desserts – non-dairy, many flavors

Cheese and Cheese Substitutes (including yogurt and creams)

If you choose to eat dairy cheese, here are some suggestions:

- Soft cheeses are healthier choices than hard cheeses. They are easier to digest, lower in fat, and contain higher quality fats and fewer chemicals. Soft cheeses are mozzarella, Brie, string, feta, ricotta and cottage cheese. Also, white or light colored cheeses are less likely to be artificially colored.
- Hard cheeses are jack, Swiss and cheddar. Hard cheeses may be more difficult to digest, therefore, more constipating than soft cheese.
- Raw and unheated cheese is more digestible than cheese that's been heated or melted. Trader Joe's and most health food stores carry raw cheeses.

Cheese Alternatives

- Follow Your Heart (soy-based: casein-free)
- The Good Slice (soy-based: contains casein) – several varieties and flavors
- HempNut Cheese Alternative (rice-based: contains casein)
- Instead O'Cheese (soy-based: casein-free) – spread
- NuTofu (soy-based: contains casein) – slices and chunks
- The Original Almond (nut-based: contains casein) - slices
- AlmondRella (nut-based; contains casein)
    - HempRella (hemp-based; contains casein)
    - TofuRella (soy-based; contains casein)
    - VeganRella (nut-based; casein-free)
    - Zero-FatRella (soy-based; contains casein)
- Smart Beat Soy Garden (soy-based, contains casein) – blocks
- Soy-Sation (soy-based, contains casein) – slices
- Soya Kaas (soy-based, contains casein) – slices, chunks, grated

- Soyco (contains casein) – Varieties of soy, almond, oat, rice – slices, chunks
- Soymage (casein-free) soy-based – singles, grated parmesan, chunk varieties
- Tofutti (soy-based, casein-free) – slices and shredded, American and mozzarella styles
- Veggie (soy-based; contains casein) – slices, grated, chunks
- Veggie Kaas (rice & oat-based, casein-free) – cheddar and mozzarella-style blocks

Cream Cheese Alternatives

- Goat cream cheese (Redwood Hill Farm Chevre)
- Rice cream cheese (Soyco)
- Soy cream cheese (Soya Kaas - contains casein)
- Vegan soy cream cheese (Soymage -casein-free)
- Soy cream cheese (Tofutti Better Than Cream Cheese - casein-free)
- Soy cream cheese and spreads (Veggie Kaas - casein-free)

Yogurt is often a good choice and can replace cheese in some dishes. With it, many sauces can be made for entrees, grains, and vegetables. The better yogurts are Alta Dena, Brown Cow, Horizon Organic, Mountain High, and Naja. Some dairy-sensitive children may be able to digest yogurt more easily, because of the enzymatic activity. Goat yogurt is also a good choice. Kefir is a yogurt drink that many kids enjoy, especially when it is fruit-sweetened.

Yogurt Substitutes

- Soygurt; all flavors
- White Wave – dairy-free, variety of flavors
- WholeSoy – dairy-free, variety of flavors

Sour Cream Alternatives

- Soyco Rice Lowfat Sour Cream Alternative
- Soymage Vegan Lowfat Sour Cream Alternative
- Tofutti Sour Supreme

Miscellaneous

- Coffee Cream - Silk Soymilk Creamer
- Parmesan Cheese - Soymage Vegan Topping, Parmesan
- Whipped Cream - Now and Zen Hip Whip

- Tofu and tempeh can be used as cheese or meat substitutes; they take different forms:
  - Soy Deli spiced tofu
  - Soy Power baked and pressed tofu
  - Wildwood Natural Foods tofu teriyaki and braised tofu chunks

Dairy-Free Meals and Entrees

- Enchiladas - vegetable, black bean varieties. Some brands contain tofu instead of cheese. (Amy's, Soypreme and Tofu Enchilada)
- Frozen lasagna - tofu filling (Legume)
- Frozen Pizza with soy cheese (Pizsoy, Farm Foods, Amy's)
- Imagine Natural Organic Soups and Broths - all varieties
- Imagine Natural Stuffed Sandwich - Indian Vegetable Curry
- Macaroni and soy cheese (frozen: Amy's)
- Manicotti or Stuffed Shells with tofu (Celentano)
- Ravioli – non-dairy varieties in your local health food store
- Stuffed shells - tofu filling (Legume)
- Szechuan Veggie Delight
- Vegetable Pot Pie

Egg Substitutes

- Egg Beaters contains egg whites, no yolks
- Ener-G Egg Replacer: This is egg-free and used most often in baking. It is best for recipes that call for 1 or 2 eggs at the most.
- Morningstar Farms - Scramblers (egg-free and gluten-free)

Wheat and Wheat-Free Foods

Whole wheat and sprouted wheat products are more nutritious for and better assimilated by the body than refined white flour products. These are easy to locate where you shop. However, many children and adults have an allergy or sensitivity to wheat or grain products. Wheat and its derivatives are found in almost every processed food, from soup to ice cream. Listed below are alternatives to wheat. I recommend that everyone rotate a variety of grain products into their diet for variety of nutrients, as well as taste.

Breads - Check store refrigerators.

- Brown rice bread (refrigerator) (Food For Life)
- Corn tortillas – yellow and blue corn (Cedarlane)
- Ener-G Tapioca Bread (made with tapioca and rice)

- Enjoy Life Bagels, gluten-free
- Essene whole rye bread (refrigerator)
- Glutino bread, many varieties, gluten-free
- Kamut bread (Oasis Bakery) – (Well-liked by kids)
- Kamut bread (Pacific Bakery)
- Manna breads (refrigerator)
- Orgran makes several gluten-free bread, muffin and stuffing mixes
- Potato bread and other mixes
- Some corn breads are wheat-free.
- Spelt bread (Rudy's, French Meadows, Food For Life, Pacific Bakery)
- Spelt tortillas (Rudy's) – white and whole spelt
- White rice bread (refrigerator) (Food For Life)
- Whole rye bread (Rudolf's, French Meadows)

Muffins

- Glutino Muffin and Scone mixes, gluten-free
- "No Muffins" is a brand name. Some are wheat-free, dairy-free and sugar-free.
- Various oat bran muffins are wheat-free
- Zen muffins - some are wheat-free

Flours - The following can be used to make wheat-free baked goods.

- Amaranth flour
- Artichoke flour
- Barley flour
- Brown rice flour
- Buckwheat flour
- Garbanzo bean flour
- Garfava flour
- Kamut flour
- Millet flour
- Oat flour and oat bran
- Potato flour
- Quinoa flour
- Spelt flour
- Sorghum
- Soy flour
- Tapioca flour
- Teff flour
- Yellow or blue corn flour

Arrowhead Mills, Bob's Red Mill, Ener-G, Miss Roben, Fearn, David Goodbatter and Pamela's all make bread, muffin, pancake, waffle and cake mixes with combinations of the above flours. Some are organic, wheat-free and/or gluten-free. Sylvan Border Farm, Bob's Red Mill and Gluten-Free Pantry produce wheat-free and gluten-free flours which are very nutritious.

Pastas – Always read the labels carefully.

- Amaranth pasta (Health Valley)
- Amy's Kids Meals, Baked Ziti (gluten-free)
- Brown rice pasta - several shapes (Pastariso)
- Corn pasta (DeBoles)
- Kamut pasta
- Mung Bean Pasta (Eden Foods)
- Noodles (Annie Chun) – rice-based
- Orgran makes 21 gluten-free pastas from rice, corn, millet and buckwheat.
- Pad Thai Noodles (Thai Kitchen, Taste of Thai)
- Quinoa pasta (Ancient Harvest, Mrs. Denson's)
- Rice elbows and other shapes (EnerG and Taste of Thai)
- Rice Lasagna (EnerG Foods)
- Rice spirals (DeBoles)
- Soba - This is buckwheat pasta and is found in the Macrobiotic or Asian sections of stores: some are 100% buckwheat and others contain a percentage of wheat. By the way, buckwheat is not a member of the wheat family!
- Spelt pasta (Purity Foods)
- Tofu Noodles (Shikataki)

Cereals – Here are healthy versions of Fruit Loops, Cheerios and many more.

- Barbara's Fruity Punch (free of wheat, dairy, chemicals)
- Fiona's All Natural Quinoa Cereal, gluten-free
- Flakes: kamut, corn, amaranth, quinoa
- Glutino's cereals
- Gorilla Munch (Enviro Kids) - great wheat-free alternative to Captain Crunch
- Kamut Krisp (Natures Path)
- Kamutios (New Morning - also like Cheerios)
- Kay Naturals Protein Cereals, gluten-free
- Muesli - This is a mixture of grains, nuts and dried fruits
- Nutty Rice (Perky's - similar to Grape Nuts)
- Oat Bran Spoonfuls (Barbara's)
- Oatios (New Morning - like Cheerios, without sugar)
- Puffed Brown Rice (Arrowhead Mills)
- Puffed Kamut (Arrowhead Mills)

All ground or flaked wheat-free grains can be used as hot cereals:

- Corn Grits (Arrowhead Mills)
- Cream of Buckwheat (Pocono)
- Cream of Rye (Roman Meal)
- Cream of Rice (Lundberg)
- Kashi (buckwheat and mixtures of other grains)
- Organic Porridge Flakes: rice and millet flakes, agar-agar (Barkat)
- Oatmeal (many brands)
- Quinoa Flakes (Ancient Harvest)
- Teff grain makes a farina-like hot cereal. (Bob's Red Mill and Maskal Teff)
- Yellow Corn

Cookies, Cakes and Bars

- Arrowhead Mills makes wheat-free and gluten-free cookie mixes.
- Barbara's – several varieties of wheat-free cookies including Fig Bars
- Clif Bar makes a kid's line called Clif Kid. It offers ZBars in various flavors. Wheat and dairy-free, organic and no trans fats. (www.clifbar.com)
- Cherrybrook Kitchen – cake mixes, free of gluten, dairy, nuts and eggs
- Ener-G - tasty varieties of wheat-free/gluten-free cookies, cakes and brownies
- Enjoy Life Soft Cookies and Snack Bars
- Fiona's Quinoa Energy Bars, (gluten-free)
- French Meadow gluten-free cookie dough and brownies
- Frookie manufactures several types of cookies, from Oreo-like to animal crackers. Since wheat may sneak into some versions, please read the labels.
- Glutino's gluten-free cookie and wafer varieties
- Health Valley – wheat-free Breakfast Bars and oatmeal cookie varieties
- Mi-Del Cookies - Choc Chip Mini's, Arrowroot Animals, Ginger Snaps (wheat-free/gluten-free)
- Newman's Own Organics Newman-O's Vanilla Cream Cookies, Chocolate Chip Cookies and Fig Newman's (wheat free/dairy free)
- Orgran - gluten and casein-free cookies, cakes, fruit bars, licorice
- Pamela's – many varieties: wheat-free, gluten-free, fruit juice-sweetened

Other

- Australian Vege Chips are made with tapioca and cassava flour.
- Blackwing Gluten-Free Jerky
- Brown Rice Crust Pizza (Natures Highlights)

- Cornmeal crust pizza
- Enjoy Life Not Nuts Mountain Combo
- Enjoy Life Chocolate Chips, free of dairy, gluten, soy, potato, sulfites
- Glutino Candy Bars, gluten-free
- Glutino Crackers, gluten-free
- Glutino Animal Cookies and Cookie Dough, gluten-free
- Glutino Donuts, gluten-free
- Glutino Pretzels and Pretzel Sticks, gluten-free
- Kay Naturals Protein Pretzels and Pretzel Sticks, gluten-free
- Kay Naturals Protein Snack Chips, Snack Mix and Kruncheeze
- Organic frozen waffles – many varieties of wheat-free (Van's, Trader Joe's and Waffle Heaven)
- Spelt Crust Pizza (Grainaissance, Nature's Highlights)

Gluten and Gluten-Free Foods

As we discussed in *Chapter 2*, the gluten issue is a controversial one, but a necessary one to understand, especially for children who have celiac disease or are gluten-sensitive. Actually, I recommend most of my patients go "gluten-free", at least most of the time. This automatically cuts many grains from the diet which is a very good thing.

What makes gluten so popular and utilized is that it makes a successful baked good, more than any other grain. It improves the "binding" and the leavening process. So, when non-gluten grains are used in baking, two or more flours are needed to make a successful product – that doesn't fall apart, isn't too dense, and doesn't taste too intense. It takes quite a bit of skill to bake gluten-free; in fact, it is an art. But it is worth developing if wheat- or gluten-containing foods are off limits to you or a family member.

Remember, a gluten allergy or sensitivity can be devastating to the digestive tract and other mucous membranes of the body. Many children and adults diagnosed with ADD, ADHD, Autistic Spectrum Disorder, celiac disease, chronic fatigue syndrome, developmental delays, diabetes, asthma and allergies must avoid gluten.

Grains and flours to AVOID by gluten-intolerant people

Barley
Bulgur
Couscous
Farina
Kasha
Oats (see *Chapter 2*)
Rye
Semolina
Spelt
Triticale

White wheat or white flour	Whole wheat

Other foods derived from or containing wheat are malt, grain starches, hydrolyzed vegetable/plant proteins, textured vegetable proteins, grain vinegars, soy sauce, grain alcohol, flavorings and the binders and fillers found in some vitamins and medications.

Gluten-Free Grains and Flours

- Amaranth - Whole grain originating back from the ancient Aztec civilization. Nutty flavor, high in protein. Use as a hot cereal, side dish or as flour.
- Arrowroot flour is used cup for cup in place of cornstarch for people who are allergic to corn.
- Buckwheat is a seed, in the rhubarb family. Groats and flour are the forms we usually see buckwheat in. Used as a side dish, hot cereal, or combined with other flours for making baked goods.
- Coconut flour – Stores well on shelf; lasts long in frig in airtight container.
- Corn flour - Flour ground from corn. Store in refrigerator or freezer.
- Corn meal - Course flour ground from corn. Stores well on shelf.
- Cornstarch - Refined starch from corn. Stores well on shelf.
- Garbanzo flour – Ground from chickpeas. Store in refrigerator or freezer.
- Garfava flour - Combination of garbanzo and fava bean flours produced by Bob's Red Mill and Authentic Foods. Stores well on shelf.
- Millet is a small, round grain originating in Africa, Asia, and India. Can be used as a side dish or hot cereal. Also milled into flour for baked goods.
- Nut flours – Used in small amounts as replacement for dry milk powder for casein-free alternative, or used to add protein to flour mixes.
- Oats – Certified gluten-free oat products from www.glutenfreeoats.com, Bob's Red Mill and www.creamhillestates.com.
- Popcorn flour - see Red cornmeal.
- Potato flour - Made from potatoes. It is not the same as potato starch. Store in refrigerator or freezer.
- Potato starch - Starch made from potatoes. Stores well on shelf.
- Quinoa – A staple food of the Incas, very high in protein. Can be used as a side dish, in salads, or milled into flour for baking. It is a high-protein grain.
- Red cornmeal - also known as popcorn flour. Stores well on shelf.
- Rice flour - Made from brown or white rice. Each one must be combined with other flours to make a successful baked good. Brown rice flour has a short shelf life and must be refrigerated. White rice flour is not as "alive".

- Sago - An easily digested form of starch, sago is derived from the pith in the trunks of the sago and other tropical palms. In the Indian grocery stores, sago is usually called "sabudhana" in Hindi, and "javvarisi" in Tamil.
- Sorghum/Jowar - Jowar is gluten and wheat free. It is a summer cereal grain that can be milled to produce starch or grits from which many ethnic & traditional dishes can be made. Stores well on shelf.
- Soy flour - Made from soybeans. Store in refrigerator or freezer.
- Sweet rice flour is made from glutinous rice, which does not contain gluten. It is often used as a thickening agent. Stores well on shelf.
- Tapioca flour/Tapioca starch - Made from cassava root. Stores well on shelf.
- Tapioca and Yucca flour combination. Cebe is the brand name.
- Teff is a grain from Ethiopia, now grown in Idaho. Difficult to sift, it is always a whole grain and high in protein. Teff is used as a cereal, in puddings and in combination with other flours for baked goods.

Most gluten-free advocate groups believe amaranth, quinoa and teff are very nutritious grains. They are rich in calcium and contain the highest amount of protein of all the grain products. A USDA survey ranked grains according to iron, protein and fiber content. Quinoa was ranked #1. Amaranth was #2.

Some people may even be sensitive to items on the list above. Perhaps they have grain allergies in general, whether gluten-containing or not. Or perhaps their reactions are to another molecule or substance in that food, or a cross-contamination issue, as discussed in *Chapter 2.*

It is up to each individual to look at the literature on these products, discuss them with your physician, and make an informed decision about their use. (See '*Resources*' in the back of the book for incredible sources of gluten-free foods.)

Meat: Meat-Free Products, Entrees and Dinners

All real meats, including beef, chicken, turkey, and seafood should be purchased from a reliable butcher shop, or natural food store such as Whole Foods, Wild Oats, Bread and Circus, Fresh Fields, Trader Joe's, Henry's, Jimbo's or your local health food store. Make sure you ask where the meat comes from, how it was produced and if it is hormone and antibiotic-free. Many stores carry free-range chicken, which means the chickens are grown in normal, out-door living conditions. These stores carry meat that is more pure than most grocery stores.

Children and adults should avoid meat that contains artificial hormones, dyes and antibiotics. These chemicals affect our immune, digestive and endocrine/hormone systems. Some even affect various functions of the brain. In light of this, it may also be interesting to try one vegetarian day a week, or one vegetarian dinner a week.

There are numerous non-animal-derived meat substitutes, mostly made from tofu, other forms of soy, wheat gluten, whole grains and mixtures of vegetables. Some of them taste astoundingly good. This is of great benefit to vegetarians and those who want to add variety to their daily diet, as well as those who are looking for another source of protein. It is vitally important, however, to read the labels, as many of these products contain foods to which your child may be sensitive or allergic. If you are trying to avoid wheat, gluten or soy, most of these products will be "off limits" to you. Many meat substitutes also contain preservatives and flavorings, so please read the labels.

Burgers

- Garden Sausage Patties (Gardenburger)
- Garden burger (made with brown rice, many varieties)
- Nature's Burger Mixes
- Tempeh burgers
- Tofu burgers (Soy Deli, Tree of Life)
- Veggie Burgers (Amy's, Natural Touch, Boca Burger, Morningstar Farms)

Frozen Dinners

- Amy's frozen dinners contain non-meat entrees with great side dishes.
- Grilled Tofu Dinners (Jaclyn)
- Salisbury Steak (meatless) Dinner (Jaclyn)
- Sirloin Strips (meatless) Dinner (Jaclyn)

Hot Dogs and Deli Slices

- Deli Slices made from gluten by Heart & Soul (turkey and roast beef style)
- Bologna or Turkey slices (Light Life/Smart Deli)
- Lean Breakfast Links (Light Life)
- Morningstar Farms also produces a wide variety of vegetarian "fake" meat products, including sausages, burgers and chicken nuggets.
- Smart Deli – various "cold cut" imitations
- Smart Dogs (regular, jumbo or spicy)
- Tofu Pups (hot dogs) by Light Life
- Tofu Wieners and Tofu Deli Slices by Yves

Other Meat Substitutes

- 5-Grain Tempeh, Sweet Brown Rice Tempeh (Grainaissance) - can be used as meat replacements in stew, chili, soup
- Falafel Mix (Fantastic Foods)
- Fillets like chicken fillets, made from soy (Hearty and Natural brand)
- Gimme Lean - veggie protein similar to ground beef
- Lemon Broil Tempeh (rice and soy-derived)
- Lentil Rice Loaf - frozen (Natural Touch)
- Nine Bean Loaf - frozen (Natural Touch)
- Smart Ground - similar to ground beef (Light Life)
- Vegetarian Chile (White Wave)
- Vegetarian Egg Rolls (White Lotus)
- Vegetarian Sloppy Joe's (White Wave)

Sugar and Its "As-Natural-As-Possible" Substitutes

Refined, white sugar, the most commonly used sweetener today, is granulated from sugar cane or from beets. Highly refined, this type of sugar is empty, containing no nutrients. For nutritional reasons, we recommend that if you eat any foods or drink any beverages with sweeteners, you would benefit by choosing from the following list.

Agave – Agave is nectar derived from the Blue agave Mexican cactus. It ranks high on the "food exchange requirements" list by the American Diabetic Association and American Dietetic Association for product labeling! Many benefits can be derived from using agave nectar as your sweetener. Agave Nectar is low calorie. It is a low glycemic food. It will not cause an over-stimulation of the production of insulin in your body. It is safe for diabetics and hypoglycemics. It does not contain processing chemicals. The nectar can be used for baking, cooking and anywhere else you would normally use sugar. It is safe and an excellent sweetener for children.

Barley malt syrup is made from sprouted barley; is a complex sweetener that's metabolized more evenly by the body. It is a thick sweetener with molasses-like flavor and dark, golden color. This sweetener offers trace amounts of B vitamins and several minerals. Use in cookies and muffins. It is one of the most balanced and unrefined sweeteners available.

Blackstrap Molasses is a bi-product if the refining process of sugar. It is dark, thick syrup, containing B vitamins and minerals such as calcium and iron. Use in ginger snaps and gingerbread.

Brown rice syrup is a traditional Asian sweetener, high in maltose and complex carbohydrates. It is absorbed more slowly into the bloodstream producing less fluctuation in blood sugar levels and mood swings than many other sweeteners. It contains trace amounts of vitamin B and minerals and is a mildly-sweet, caramel-colored syrup, similar to honey in consistency. It is best used in puddings and toppings.

Cane sugar syrup is simply unrefined cane juice boiled down to syrup; in much the same way that maple syrup is produced.

Date sugar is a concentrated sweetener from dried and ground dates, which retains most of the vitamins and minerals found in dates. It is high in fiber and contains a wide variety of vitamins and minerals.

Florida Crystals is dehydrated sugar cane juice containing more minerals than white, refined sugar, but it is still sugar. Use cup for cup in any recipe that calls for sugar.

Fruit Source is made from a natural blend of grapes and rice carbohydrates. It replaces both the sugar and the fat in baking. To use in baking, replace every cup of sugar with 1 1/4 cups Fruitsource and reduce fat by 50%. Do not exceed 325° F degrees in baking.

Fructo-oligosaccharides (FOS) is a natural sugar. Found in powder form, this food primarily comes from Jerusalem artichokes, chicory, asparagus and soybeans. NuNaturals makes a good product.

Fructose is utilized in granulated and syrup forms and is almost twice as sweet as white sugar. The difference is, it releases glucose into the bloodstream more slowly than white sugar, making it safer for some people with blood sugar imbalances. Others, however, are just as sensitive to fructose as they are to white, refined sugar or sucrose. There is little nutritional value in fructose.

Fruit juice concentrates are often used in cookies and muffins. Thaw frozen juice concentrates and use in place of sugar.

Honey comes in hundreds of varieties depending on the flower that produces them. For the highest quality of beneficial enzymes and nutrients, choose raw, unpasteurized honey. Sweet and golden, it is excellent in cakes, cookies and muffins.

Luo Han Guo is syrup from a fruit grown in China, containing mogrosides which are 300 times sweeter than sucrose, fructose or glucose. It is not really a sugar and has demonstrated in research to not cause insulin levels to rise. It is low calorie and natural, but has a bit of an aftertaste.

Maple sugar is made by boiling maple syrup to evaporate the liquid. It is about twice as sweet as white sugar. Make sure you buy organic versions, as some producers use formaldehyde to increase the flow of sap. It tastes great on hot cereals.

Maple syrup is less viscous than honey and is extracted from the maple tree. It is highly nutritious, especially when fresh, containing B vitamins and minerals. Grades B and C are darker and stronger-tasting than Grade A, and therefore more mineral-rich. Use in cookies, cakes and muffins, over pancakes or straight off the spoon.

SlimSweet is derived from a medicinal Chinese fruit of the kiwi family and is a natural sweetener similar to fructose, but without the calories. SlimSweet contains zero calories per 1 gram serving and is a thermogenic (fat-burning) substance as well. SlimSweet tastes just like sugar but is 15 times as sweet. One-fifth teaspoon is equal to 3 teaspoons of sugar. SlimSweet has a low glycemic index, which means it does not significantly elevate blood sugar or insulin levels.

Sorghum Syrup is produced in the same manner as cane syrup, but sorghum cane, rather than sugar cane, is used. Sorghum tends to have a thinner, slightly-more sour taste than cane syrup.

Stevia is a South American herb originating in Paraguay, 100 to 400 times sweeter than white sugar. It is calorie-free, doesn't upset blood sugar levels, and can actually help regulate them. Available as a greenish powder, stevia imparts an intense sweetness with an herbal undertone. As sweeteners go, it may appear to be expensive, but a little goes a long way. Liquid or powder form, it is great to use in liquids, tea and coffee, or to dissolve in any milk before you put it on cereal.

Steviva Blend is a blend of the highest quality stevia extract and erythritol, a filler which is naturally-occurring in a variety of foods and derived from fermented glucose. Steviva Blend is granulated like sugar and dissolves quickly. It has a 1:1 sweetness ratio to sugar, so it is very easy to measure. It is ideal for baking and cooking. Steviva Blend has less than 1 calorie and less than 1 gram carbohydrate per serving, making it safe for diabetics. It may be used in hot or cold liquids or sprinkled on cereals and fruit.

Sucanat is evaporated cane juice and consists of fine ground brown crystals, with a mild molasses flavor. It substitutes cup for cup in baked goods and is extremely versatile. Darker than most cane sugar, it contains more nutrients, especially minerals.

Sugar Alcohols – *Arabitol, Erythritol, Glycerol, Isomalt, Lactitol, Malitol, Maltitol, Mannitol, Sorbitol, Xylitol* are all polyols or sugar alcohols. Though derived from fruits and vegetables such as corn and birch tree fiber, these sweeteners are not really “natural”. They are manufactured by the fermentation of glucose and have a caloric value of close to zero. Nearly as sweet as sucrose, the sugar alcohols are used cup for cup, like sugar. With no after-taste, they can be used to make sugar-free, no-sugar- added or reduced-calorie bakery goods. They have no nutritional value. They are slowly absorbed and have a low-glycemic value, making them desirable for diabetics. Because of the slow absorption, however, the sugar alcohols may cause gas, bloating and diarrhea, especially if consumed in large amounts.

Turbinado Sugar is made from cane juice or from sugar beets. It is a light tan color with shiny crystals from whole sugar cane, with slightly (but not much) more trace nutrients than refined white sugar.

Zero or Zsweet both look like, flow and taste like sugar. Use 1:1 like sugar. ZSweet is a blend of erythritol and natural flavor enhancement and Zero is only erythritol. They are neither chemically-altered, nor herbal extracts. They provide zero calories and are made by fermentation not hydrogenation. They are a little less sweet than sugar. On the down side, they may cause gas, bloating or diarrhea.

Sweeteners for Cereals

- Agave syrup
- Barley malt – syrup-like molasses (Eden)
- Brown rice syrup

- Florida Crystals - mineral-rich, from sugar cane
- FOS (fructoligosaccharides)
- Honey - raw (Do not use for children under age 2.)
- Maple syrup - unprocessed, pure, grade A or B
- Molasses (Plantain) – strong flavor due to its mineral content
- Maple sugar
- SlimSweet
- Sucanat - pure, granulated sugar cane (mineral-rich)
- Stevia - liquid (Planetary Formulas) or powder. Dissolve in liquid before putting it on cereal.
- Xylitol – granulated sugar alcohol which is a low-glycemic substitute for sugar
- Zsweet or Zero - substitute 1:1 for sugar

Sweeteners for Drinks

- Apple concentrate can be added to sparkling or non-sparkling water.
- Black cherry concentrate (Hain)
- Chocolate beverage products: Organic chocolate syrup sweetened with cane juice made by Ah Alaska and Santa Cruz. Hot chocolate, 99.7% caffeine free and sweetened with SlimSweet, made by Wonderslim. Chocolate agave syrup found at www.realfoodtrading.com.
- Cranberry concentrate (Hain)
- Grape juice concentrate (Cascadian Farms)
- Stevia is available in liquid (Sunrider, Planetary Formulas, Now) or powder. The liquid form is excellent in hot and iced herbal teas, sparkling water and smoothies.
- Xylitol
- Zsweet or Zero

Sweeteners for Baking

- Brown rice syrup can be used alone or in combination with maple syrup, as it is only mildly sweet.
- Fruit juice concentrates (grape, black cherry and apple) can be used in baking, but some people are clearly sensitive to them.
- Honey can be used in many recipes but has a distinctive flavor because of the high mineral content.
- Maple syrup is good for baking but also has a distinctive flavor. Use the real thing, not commercial grocery store brands.

- Sucanat, or pure granulated sugar cane, substitutes cup for cup in baking. Because of its color, however, it will darken all baked goods.
- Xylitol – very successful in baking
- Zsweet or Zero – substitute cup for cup, a little less sweet than sugar.

Other Baking Needs

- Check www.naturesflavors.com for organic fruit syrups, concentrates, organic food-based flavor extracts and food-based food colorings derived from fruits and vegetables.
- Suzanne's Rice Mellow – marshmallow, free of gluten and dairy

Spreads, Nut Butters and Much More

Fresh cut vegetables, crackers, rice cakes or baked chips may be used with many fine tasting spreads which are healthy and appropriate for allergic and sensitive children. Fresh, raw peanut butter can be bought at many health food stores. Commercial peanut butters are high in fat and sugar. They are a poor quality food to which many children are allergic. Peanuts (a legume) may contain a very harmful mold, called aflatoxin. Here are some alternatives:

- Almond butter tastes similar to peanut butter and is a more digestible protein.
- Cashew butter is also tasty, creamy nut butter.
- Hazelnut butter
- Macadamia butter
- Walnut butter
- Hummus or garbanzo bean dip can be used as a spread or to fill a pita.
- Tahini or sesame butter are good spreads, high in calcium & vitamin E.
- Justin's Nut Butters are sold in convenient single serving packets.
- Dips can be used as spreads: black bean dip, pinto bean dip, artichoke, etc.
- Jellies and jams: Trader Joe's and most health food stores carry healthier jellies and jams than most grocery stores. Use fruit juice-sweetened. Some brand names are Sorrell Ridge, Whole Foods, L&A and Knudsen.
- Instead of margarine, use raw or organic butter, Horizon or Organic Valley.
- A wonderful non-dairy butter substitute is Earth's Balance Buttery Spread. It contains no GMO's, trans-fatty acids or casein.
- Spectrum Naturals Spreads substitute for butter. They are dairy-free, with non- hydrogenated oils; available in Olive and Mediterranean varieties.

- Try your favorite olive oil with a little sea salt on toast, vegetables or baked potato.
- Mayonnaise - Good-tasting mayo's and sandwich spreads:
    - Vegenaise – Egg-free and made with grape seed oil
    - Nayonaise – Egg-free
    - Spectrum Naturals - Excellent quality oils and mayonnaise

---

1. *Haenlein, George, F.W, Extension Goat Handbook, University of Delaware, and Donald L. Ace, Pennsylvania State University*

~ ~ ~

Chapter Ten

EASY MEALS
Don't Drive Yourself Crazy

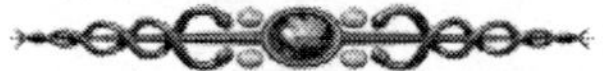

Problems & Solutions to Eating on School Days

I'm sure you can relate – not hungry in the morning? It's not always easy to get our kids to have a good breakfast so early in the day. There are time constraints and physiological constraints. But there are ways to strike a happy medium. It is so important to fuel the brain on a regular basis, especially after having fasted overnight. Breakfast time is truly a time for breaking the fast and starting the day with good fuel.

1. Our children are not eating breakfasts that support proper brain function. They are not taking in the proper nutrients to manufacture the brain chemicals or neurotransmitters. For this they need proportionally balanced and easily assimilable proteins, essential fatty acids, trace minerals and complex carbohydrates.

Possible effects of an "un-fueled" brain:

- hyperactivity
- lack of focus and attention
- poor memory
- foggy thinking
- day-dreaming
- depression
- poor hand-eye coordination
- grouchy, irritable, mood swings

The following study states that omitting breakfast interferes with learning, cognition and school performance. Also noted in this particular study, when breakfast is consumed, school attendance and the quality of the students' diets improve.

Breakfast and Cognition: An Integrative Summary
Pollitt E; Mathews R, *American Journal of Clinical Nutrition* 1998 Apr; 67(4):804S-813S (98196983 NLM)

The pooled data suggests that omitting breakfast interferes with cognition and learning, an effect that is more pronounced in nutritionally at-risk children than in well-nourished children. Breakfast consumption improves school attendance, reduces tardiness and enhances the quality of the students' diets.

2. Our children are not eating the type of breakfasts that stabilize blood sugar. Again, for this they need proportionally balanced and easily assimilable protein, fatty acids, trace minerals and complex carbohydrates.

Possible effects of blood sugar imbalance:

- irritability
- mood swings
- foggy thinking
- aggressive behavior
- energy dips, fatigue sets in easily
- cravings for sugar or stimulants

The cravings for sugar or stimulant foods such as coffee and caffeinated sodas sometimes resemble that of an addict. "I gotta have it now" is how the behavior is translated. The brain needs the fuel; the body needs the fuel, the quickest way possible. I have heard more than once from moms that they catch their child kneeling on the kitchen counter pouring sugar into his or her mouth, straight from the bag. Sometimes when you need the fuel, you "gotta have it now". Unfortunately, poor choices are made out of desperation.

3. Our children are not eating the type of breakfasts that fuel the adrenal glands in order to balance stress and produce enough energy to carry out their mental and physical activities. Once again, for this they need proportionally balanced and easily assimilated proteins, fatty acids, trace minerals and complex carbohydrates.

Possible effects of low adrenal function:

- lack of focus and concentration
- fatigue
- poor sleep habits: restless sleep or difficulty in waking
- sluggish bowel function – tend toward constipation (less than 2 bowel movements per day)
- decreased athletic abilities
- lack of focus and concentration during athletic practices or games
- proneness to sedentary lifestyle: excess T.V. and video watching and computer game playing
- lowered metabolism, leading to obesity

Childhood obesity is now at a raging 25%. One quarter of all children in America is overweight. Obesity may result at an early age or later in life due to:

- the inability to sustain the necessary energy to carry out normal childhood physical activities or perform in athletics on any level
- attraction to sedentary activities such as watching television or playing computer games

4. Some children are not eating breakfast at all. They are getting no fuel for the brain or the body. This is a severe problem. The next study from the *American Journal of Clinical Nutrition* indicates that consumption of food, beverage or both at breakfast has decreased especially in teenagers, at least 15-20%. It was noted that only 64.7% of girls ages 15-18 eat breakfast. A large percent of children do not consume breakfast and a general decrease was noted in children of all ages. An obvious association exists between decreased breakfast consumption and obesity, as there has been rise in obesity in children over age 11. Here is the study:

Trends in Breakfast Consumption for Children in the United States
Siega-Riz AM; Popkin BM; Carson T, *Amer Journal Clini Nutr*, 1998 Apr; 67(4):748S-756S (98196974 NLM)

"We examined breakfast consumption patterns and trends for children (1-10 yr old) and adolescents (11-18 yr old) in the U.S. **Results indicated a decline in breakfast consumption, 15% in boys and 20% in girls**, particularly for older adolescents. A large percentage of children aged 11 and over do not consume breakfast. "Given the association of **obesity** with less frequent breakfast consumption and the rise in obesity in this age group, a renewed emphasis on the importance of breakfast is warranted."

Again, we have a serious problem here. And you know it's largely the fault of the system. Up at 6 a.m. and in your seat by 7:40 is the reality. We tend to scold our children consistently at this time of day. We may feel guilty for sending them off without the proper nutrients and fuel to sustain good academic performance, good behavior, good attitudes and good energy.

And the funny thing is, we as adults, do the same. A cup of coffee and a donut or scone is a typical example of the breakfast of many working parents. Are we presenting ourselves as good examples?

No. Is it our fault? No, not completely. Who is to blame? Everyone. We created, uphold and support the system by not changing it. Change is best made at the grass roots level. **The solutions begin at home and in the**

classroom. In the last chapter of this book, you will find ideas about "*What Parents Can Do*" and "*What Teachers Can Do*" to make these changes.

So, we know that breakfast is important. Whether it's cereal, a smoothie or eggs, the human body needs fuel after its nightly fast. From roughly 9:00 PM to 7:00 AM, most adults and children are not eating. They are relaxing or sleeping; they are fasting. Breakfast breaks that fast in order to fuel the body and brain tissues and start the new day. In the following pages you will find ideas from quick, out-the-door breakfast foods, to traditional and weekend breakfast ideas.

Power Breakfasts

- Upon arising, drink 6-8 ounces of fresh, pure water.
- Fruit juice should be kept to a minimum, but when consumed, should be diluted with water by one third.
- 1-2 scrambled or over-easy eggs. 1 small red potato sautéed into hash browns.
- 1-2 scrambled eggs, wrapped in a corn tortilla. Side of fruit.
- Whole grain toast or bagel with almond or cashew butter and fruit-sweetened jam or raw honey.
- 1-2 whole grain or gluten-free waffles with cinnamon sugar (made with sugar substitute such as Sucanat) or raw honey or honeycomb.
- 2 whole grain or gluten-free pancakes. (See *Healthy Substitutes List* for suggested mixes.) Top with ground sunflower, flax or sesame seeds and pure maple syrup or fruit sweetened jam.
- Fruit smoothie. (See *Smoothie* section for options.)
- Whole grain muffin. (See *Healthy Substitutes List* for options.) Add a side dish of yogurt.
- 1 cup whole grain cold cereal with organic dairy milk, rice milk, Van's Dairy Free or almond milk. Use alternative natural sweetener, if desired. (See *Healthy Substitutes List.*)
- Whole grain hot cereal such as: oatmeal, cream of buckwheat, cream of rice, or kashi with honey or stevia to sweeten, and rice milk, hemp milk or dairy milk.
- Brown rice pudding with raisins or dried dates and rice or dairy milk. For sweetener use stevia, honey or maple syrup, not refined sugar. (Can be made a day ahead.)
- Yogurt with fresh, sliced blueberries, strawberries or banana.

Helpful Hints:

1. If your child does not like eggs, you can add ground sesame and sunflower seeds to a pancake breakfast (on top or in the batter) for protein and essential fatty acids.
2. Sugar, honey or maple syrup should not be used daily. But if you use maple syrup, you can pre-dilute the maple syrup with flax oil for extra essential fatty acids. This will typically go undetected.
3. Who says we have to only eat breakfast food in the morning. And – no – I don't mean pizza! A bowl of a favorite, piping hot soup on a cold morning may hit the spot. Maybe a piece of sliced turkey or ½ a burger from the night before. There are so many non-breakfast options to choose from. All it takes is for the light to go on – a shift in perception – to eat "outside the box".

Quick "Out-the-Door" Breakfasts

- Sliced organic turkey
- Apple, banana or other piece of fruit
- Trail mix (if not allergic to nuts)
- Whole grain breakfast bar, such as Clif Kid ZBar, organic, wheat and dairy-free, no trans fats
- Organic yogurt (Maple and vanilla are better choices than fruit-sweetened)
- Fruit smoothie with rice or whey protein
- Hemp, rice or whey protein shake with organic dairy milk, goat milk or rice milk
- Cottage cheese with ground sunflower and flax seeds

Protein Smoothies and Shakes

The majority of protein smoothies on the market are soy, whey or rice protein. They all taste fairly good, depending on the sweeteners used. Many kids like them; some don't. If your child is sensitive or allergic to soy or whey, as they are common allergens, a hemp-based or rice-based protein smoothie would be a better choice. Hemp protein is an excellent source of essential fatty acids.

Whey is an excellent source of protein and not as allergenic as soy. Two types of whey are available commercially: cow whey and goat whey. Cow whey is a dairy product, but is generally well-tolerated by dairy-sensitive individuals. It can be added to rice or almond and whipped up with an ice cube, like a milk shake. It is astoundingly tasty.

Goat whey is even better for most dairy-sensitive individuals. It is highly absorbable and contains the important electrolyte minerals. It can be used before or after school, or during or after athletic games. You can buy whey protein powder at most health food stores, but watch for artificial sweeteners on the label. (Consult the *What to Avoid List* in *Chapter 2.)*

In fact, you might add some stevia sweetener (natural sweetener from the stevia plant) because some whey shakes do not contain much, if any, sugar. The added rice, hemp, or almond milk can provide extra early morning protein to feed your child's (and your own!) neurotransmitters and expedite better focus and concentration. No mid-morning slumps!

Also, if your child just isn't up for eating or drinking anything in the morning, you can put his or her shake or smoothie into a sports bottle or thermos and they can drink it later, when they are ready.

Fruit and Juice Smoothies

Many children love fruit smoothies, especially with bananas and/or berries. It is best to start with fresh squeezed juice, squeezed or extracted in your own kitchen. If you don't have the time, most health food stores and many grocery stores sell fresh juices in their refrigerators. Some even have fresh juice bars.

Next best is the organic juice in bottles on the shelves in your health food store or grocery store. Many children look forward to freezing their banana for their smoothie the next day. The banana adds a thick consistency that works well when there is no protein powder added. Berries provide vitamins, minerals and all those little seeds that pass their life quality on to us. On top of that, they are gorgeous and can turn a thick, muddy smoothie into a fantastic red, pink, purple or lavender. If organic berries are not in season or available, there are several companies that provide them frozen in bags. Most health food stores carry them and some grocery stores do as well.

A Great Disguise for Nutritional Supplements

All smoothies and shakes can provide a medium for powder or liquid nutritional supplements. Even the contents of capsules can be opened and 'snuck' into a smoothie or shake. Digestive enzymes, acidophilus and bifidus capsules, or any other necessary nutrient in capsule or powder form, can be easily and disguisably blended into the liquid breakfast.

Dark, intensely-colored strawberry, blueberry, carob or chocolate shakes and smoothies successfully allow children to drink their breakfast containing the nutrient rich, blue green algae without noting a color change. Any green food can be disguised with the right color. Funny, how many kids think green is gross. It may take a period of adjustment and a shift of "what they're used to" for some kids, as well as parents. Since smoothies are sweet, most children adapt. Here are some kid-tested recipes:

Joe Jo's Pink Surprise

- 8 ounces any red juice (naturally red cherry cider, raspberry, cranberry)
- 1 scoop dairy whey, goat whey, hemp, rice or other protein powder
- 2 teaspoons of lecithin powder
- 1 teaspoon of any organic, cold-pressed oil: flax, hemp, fish or favorite essential fatty acid oil
- ½ cup frozen strawberries or other berries
- ½ frozen banana
- 2 ice cubes
- ¼ cup water
- Can add ½ cup yogurt as desired

Blend and drink. This mixture hides, very nicely, any supplements, even the green ones, derived from algae or barley grass.

Are You Sure There's No Ice Cream in This?

- 12 ounces vanilla or chocolate rice, hemp or almond milk (or dairy milk, if not allergic)
- If using plain or vanilla milk, you can add 1 tsp. organic cocoa powder
- 2 tablespoons whey, goat whey, hemp or rice protein powder
- 1 teaspoon of lecithin powder
- 10-15 drops of liquid stevia or equivalent stevia powder (or other natural sweetener)
- 2 ice cubes

You can add a greens powder or blue green algae capsules. They will be camouflaged. Blend and serve.

Chocolate or Vanilla Shake

- 8 ounces plain milk of choice – goat, dairy, rice, coconut or mixture
- ½ tsp vanilla or 1 tsp. cocoa powder or 2 tsp. chocolate agave syrup
- 1 tablespoon almond butter or organic peanut butter
- 2 ice cubes
- 1 tablespoon Lean Body Whey protein powder
- 2 teaspoons of lecithin powder
- Can add liquid stevia to taste (or other natural sweetener)

Blend until smooth and creamy. (This is good medium for any supplements, green food powder, blue green algae or barley green. The chocolate, the nut butter and the banana all cover any strong taste.)

Super Pina Colada Smoothie

- ½ cup pineapple coconut juice
- 2 cups rice, almond or dairy milk
- 1 ripe banana (use frozen banana to cut down on ice needed)
- 2 tablespoons whey or rice protein powder or other smoothie mix
- 1 teaspoon of lecithin powder

The Winning Combination

- 1 banana
- ½ cup frozen blueberries, strawberries or other berries
- 1 tablespoon whey, hemp, rice or other protein powder
- 8 ounces goat or rice milk
- 1 tablespoon flax oil (or other therapeutic oil)
- 1 tablespoon Tocotriene powder (rice bran and antioxidant)
- 1 teaspoon lecithin powder

Blend and serve. Serves two.

Energy or Protein Bars

There are numerous protein/energy bars on the market. The ones without refined sugar and dairy products are the best. Some energy bars are notorious for containing hidden additives and trans fats. Read labels very carefully when shopping for these snack foods.

Some companies manufacture energy bars derived from whole grains, without hidden sugar and additives. Clif Bar has a variety of bars for children called Clif Kid ZBars. They are organic, wheat and dairy-free and contain no trans fats.

Power Lunches: School and Home

Lunch is perhaps the most important meal of the day for many children. The early morning rush doesn't always allow enough time for kids to eat a well-rounded breakfast. Some children are not hungry in the morning. This puts the burden of most of the day's nutritional intake on the lunch meal.

Think about it. Kids of all ages have to meet their academic demands, social demands, and physical/athletic demands with the nutrition that they take in at breakfast and lunch. If breakfast is scanty, lunch needs to be power-packed.

A power-packed lunch is best achieved if the child or teenager brings a homemade lunch to school. You will have more control over the quality and balance of nutrients in the meal. The older the children get, the more difficult it is to convince them of this. Buying lunch at school is more socially acceptable. Unfortunately, most school lunches do not offer the comprehensive array of nutrients needed by growing children.

Even if your kids buy lunch at school, send them off with healthy snacks. Baked potato chips, low-fat granola bars, cut-up veggies and fruit are good choices. Put the food into super-hero lunch bags or a container that is appealing to them.

Power Lunch Ideas

Choose your child's favorite veggies and put them in their lunch box daily. The following ideas are designed for school lunches as well as for weekends or other days at home.

- Black bean burrito with salad.
- Chicken tostada salad with lettuce, tomatoes.
- PB&J - There is such a thing as a healthy peanut butter and jelly sandwich Use whole grain or gluten-free bread with natural peanut butter (without sugar) or almond butter and a fruit-sweetened jelly. There are many versions.
- Baked potato with steamed broccoli or other vegetables or green salad.
- Salmon or tuna salad sandwich. Use whole grain or gluten free bread, and put fresh vegetables inside: lettuce, tomato, sprouts, carrots, cucumber.
- Sliced turkey or chicken sandwich on whole grain bread with a healthy mayo and lettuce. Choose a meat that is free of hormones, antibiotics and nitrites.
- Vegetable sandwich with tomato, cucumber, lettuce, sprouts, avocado, shredded carrots or any favorite vegetables. Use organic cream cheese, goat cheese or tofu versions.
- Homemade chicken noodle or minestrone soup in a thermos and a half favorite sandwich.
- Meatloaf sandwich (beef, turkey, lentil or bean loaf) lettuce and a natural mayo on whole grain, spelt, kamut or rice bread.
- Use leftovers from dinner the night before: muffins, soup and chicken.
- Broiled chicken strips with roasted red potatoes and broccoli.
- Salmon patty, turkey burger, or veggie burger on whole grain bread with mayo or mustard, lettuce, tomato.
- Cucumber and cream cheese sandwich on whole grain or gluten-free bread.
- Hard-boiled egg, fresh cut carrots, celery and cucumber with almond or cashew butter or favorite dip.

- Organic hot dogs (nitrite-free) or tofu dogs with baked beans (put in thermos.)
- Make a sandwich more appealing by using toasted frozen waffles, whole grain or the gluten-free variety.
- Organic grilled cheese on whole grain or gluten-free bread, with grilled tomato and red onion. (For dairy allergic children, use goat, rice or soy cheese.)

Beverage Options (for school and home lunches)

- Spring water or other pure water. Best option.
- Rice milk (in little aseptic boxes, as above.)
- Natural juice
- Herbal iced teas, sweetened with stevia extract or FOS powder are very refreshing.
- Herb tea and fruit juice mixed
- Fruit smoothie in a sports bottle or thermos
- Protein shake in goat, rice, soy or whey in a sports bottle or thermos

Smart Snacks

On the run? Choose from this list. Many are appropriate for the car, plane, backpack or suitcase:

1. Green drink of choice – can bring the powder and just shake into a water bottle as desired. Simplexity Go Green has a great taste, as do Nano Greens.
2. Clear Vite or rice protein shake in water, rice, hemp or almond milk
3. Hemp protein shake (add to rice or almond milk)
4. Whey protein powder in rice, almond or hemp milk
5. ½ - 1 Cardio Pro bar, lemon-poppy seed or chocolate
6. Clif Kids ZBar
7. 3-6 oz. organic goat, dairy, soy, almond or rice milk (can pack)
8. ½ cup of organic dairy or goat yogurt
9. Cottage cheese (can add ground sesame, sunflower or flax seeds)
10. Handful sunflower seeds, pumpkin seeds, pine nuts
11. Handful almonds, walnuts or Brazil nuts, raw (can salt yourself)
12. Carrot and celery sticks with nut butter, almond or cashew, or tahini
13. ½ - 1 apple, sliced with a handful (8-12) almonds
14. ½ cup plain yogurt with 2 tablespoons blueberries
15. 2 rice or Akmak crackers with almond or cashew butter, or tahini
16. Whole grain oat cakes or rice crackers with favorite cheese or goat cheese

17. 2-3 oz. tuna salad or salmon salad
18. 2-3 oz. chicken salad
19. 2-3 oz. egg salad or 1 hard-boiled egg
20. Turkey or turkey bacon, rolled in large lettuce leaf with favorite dressing
21. Miso soup - from paste or instant travel packet (Edwards & Sons)
22. Lentil soup, black bean or other bean soup
23. 3 bean salad (sugar free, make with honey or brown rice syrup)
24. Vegetarian options: tofu hot dog, ½ veggie burger, ½ tempeh burger
25. ½ all beef or turkey hot dog, organic
26. ¼ - ½ cup cooked amaranth or quinoa cereal and rice or almond milk
27. ¼ - ½ cup cream of buckwheat/oatmeal, add ground sesame or flax seeds
28. Beanit Butter – soy butter
29. Gluten-free Rice thins or Multigrain with buckwheat thins – Trader Joe's
30. Blackwing Gluten-Free Jerky
31. Enjoy Life Foods – Mountain Mambo Gluten Free, Nut-Free Trail Mix
32. Glutino – Gluten-free pretzels
33. Apple, banana, grapes, cooked sweet potato

Family Dinners

A Harvard Medical School study on the eating habits of 16,000 children found that the kids who ate dinner with their families consumed more fruits and vegetables, fewer fried foods and more fiber than those who rarely ate with their folks. Why? First, meals at home tend to have less fat, salt and sugars than fast food restaurant meals. Second, there is more closeness among family members when time is taken to sit and eat together.

The following meal suggestions are designed to be appealing to the whole family. Alter where you would like, if making substitutions for your children.

The Basic Meal

- Crusted, broiled chicken strips or broiled or baked turkey
- Side dish: potatoes – baked or mashed or steamed brown rice (Serve with butter or olive oil and herbs.)
- Mixed green salad or steamed green vegetable of choice

A Little Bit of Italy

- Spaghetti (whole grain or wheat-free with tomato sauce, pesto sauce or butter
- Beef or turkey or veggie meatballs
- Mixed green salad
- Whole grain or wheat-free garlic bread, with olive oil and chopped garlic

Baked Oven Favorites

- Oven fried chicken
- Baked macaroni and cheese
- Green peas

Baked Potato Bar

- Add any toppings the family likes: organic butter, cheese or sour cream, onions, chives, tomatoes, broccoli, bacon and anything else?
- Put all the toppings on the table, so everyone can choose his or her own.

Loafing at Home

- Meatloaf using turkey, ground beef or lentils
- Mashed potatoes and gravy
- Steamed broccoli

Deli Stop – special weekend meal

- Sub sandwiches with whole grain bread, organic turkey or roast beef, lettuce, tomato, onion, organic pickles
- Organic baked "French fries"

Light and Lively

- Homemade chunky vegetable soup (with alphabet pasta)
- Caesar salad with chicken
- Whole grain crackers or rice cakes with almond, peanut or cashew butter

South of the Border Taco Bar – assemble your own

- Organic refried beans, organic tacos, shredded lettuce, diced tomato, shredded cheese, organic sour cream, guacamole
- Can add cooked ground organic turkey or ground beef

Omega Delight

- Salmon, broiled with lemon dill sauce
- Steamed carrots and zucchini
- Favorite muffin recipe

Malt Shop Night

- Hamburgers or cheeseburgers (ground turkey or beef) or bean burgers
- Homemade baked potato skins or organic frozen French fries
- Lettuce, tomatoes, onions, pickles (organic is best)
- Spelt, gluten free or other whole grain buns

Asian Delight

- Stir-fried chicken nuggets
- Bok choy, broccoli, snow peas, celery, onions steamed or stir-fried
- Wok-fried brown rice with sesame oil (add egg, if desired)

Fast Break Omelet Dinner

- Omelets (good place to hide veggies)
- Mashed potatoes or organic homemade hash browns
- Mixed baby green salad or romaine with favorite salad dressing

Round the Table

- Pizza: Purchase the pizza crust from a local pizza restaurant. Make at home and let the kids choose the toppings. Rice crust, cornmeal crust or spelt crust pizzas are available from the frozen foods section of most health food stores, for those with allergies.
- Mixed green salad

Winter Warmth

- Beef, turkey or vegetarian chile
- Tossed green salad with favorite dressing
- Corn bread

Suggestions and Shortcuts for Family Dinners

1. Always include at least 2 vegetables at night, either in salad, steamed or sautéed. Steaming and sautéing are the best ways to cook vegetables to preserve the nutrient values and enhance their digestibility and fibrous effect on the body.
2. Alternate your grains. Use wheat or gluten-free pasta one night, brown rice the next, corn bread the next, etc.
3. Alternate your meat products as well. Use organic and free-range versions of chicken and turkey. Rotate with varieties of deep-sea fish. Beef is O.K. upon occasion, but must be hormone-free. Cut out pork altogether. (This includes chops, hot dogs, ham, bacon, sausage.)

4. Soups are often meals in themselves. Include a salad and a slice of your homemade whole grain bread.
5. Grains and meats can be used the next day for lunch if you have leftovers.
6. Soups and casseroles can be made in large quantities and frozen in portions. Thaw out as needed for night-time meals.
7. Avoid eating fruit with a meal, as it may cause gas or bloating.
8. Water or herb teas (iced or hot) should be the only beverages with dinner. If homework is going to follow, it is best to avoid any sweet drinks that might throw off the child's blood sugar level. Balance of the blood sugar will ensure better concentration, moods, attitudes and behavior.

Also, it is observed by many parents that drinking milk or sodas with a meal decreases the child's appetite for real food.

What If My Child Won't Eat or Isn't Hungry?

1. If the child is on medication, especially a stimulant medication that causes suppression of the appetite, wait until his or her appetite returns, when the medication affect has worn off. Offer them a snack with the family at mealtime and a full meal later. Honor the body.
2. Eliminate the cause: If the medication is known to suppress the appetite, ask the doctor to switch to another medication (for ADHD, for example) that doesn't cause appetite suppression.
3. Present the food in pretty and colorful ways. Consider changing the shapes of the portions.
4. Encourage the child to try one new food per week, with "just one bite".
5. Experiment with a variety of foods – crunchy, creamy, chewy, sweet, salty, spicy, and sour to find out what the child likes and encourage him or her with options.
6. Make it a liquid meal --- a smoothie or a sweet fresh-squeezed fruit juice with carrot and celery added. Call it a milkshake. Kids relate better to that. (So do adults!)
7. Consider "trickle feeding". (Thank you, Dr. John Taylor.) Offer small amounts of food incrementally. Use the Protein Snack List in this book.
8. Involve the child in the meal planning and food preparation.
9. Eliminate milk, soda and juice. These are really foods and they are filling! Use water and herb teas. (Herb iced tea sweetened with stevia tastes great!)
10. Investigate whether your child's sense of taste or smell are decreased or lost, thus contributing to poor appetite. Some medications can cause this, as well as nutrient deficiencies of B12 or zinc. There is a simple zinc taste

test that can be done with a special zinc liquid, which tastes like water if you are deficient. If you're not, it will taste horrible! Many kids, especially those with ADHD have zinc deficiencies. (Call 800-608-5602 for the zinc taste test.) Replenishing the nutrient deficiencies helps restore the sense of taste and smell.

11. If the child is constantly battling congestion (sinus or nasal), the sense of taste or smell may become distorted or lost. When chronic congestion is cleared up, by eliminating allergy foods and improving immune function, the sense of taste or smell is often restored and the appetite returns.
12. Digestive discomfort such as gas, bloating, cramping, acid reflux, constipation and diarrhea are sometimes difficult for children to communicate about. A natural response is to avoid food. Do some detective work to see if this is the problem.
13. Keep mealtime conversations light and relaxing. (I know it's hard sometimes!) Play soft music in the background.

~ ~ ~

Chapter Eleven

SPECIAL DIETS FOR SPECIAL CHILDREN

Millions of children in North America have been diagnosed with a medical condition – a physical or a mental disease. Most of them are taking prescription medications of one kind or another, but their doctors are not telling their parents what to feed them. That's because they don't know; they haven't been taught that food can make an impact on or assist in turning around symptoms and diseases. This chapter is intended to do just that – bring to light, specific diets and food programs which are beneficial to children with pre-disease conditions and special needs.

Balanced Glycemic Diet

If everyone followed this diet, we would have fewer arguments, less depression, less obesity, less coffee consumption, better sleep, high vitality and energy, and happier people. A person on a balanced glycemic diet utilizes nutritional tools, such as *glycemic index* and *glycemic load* to balance their blood sugar. These are categories that carbohydrates, fruits, grains, sugars and starches are put in.

A balanced glycemic diet helps to normalize a "roller coaster" blood sugar effect, physically and mentally. This can greatly impact physical and mental energy. This diet can be very helpful for children with the following conditions:

- ADD
- ADHD
- Autism
- Behavior disorders
- Bi polar disorder
- Depression
- Developmental delays
- Diabetes (Type 1 and 2)
- Dyslexia
- Hypoglycemia
- Insulin resistance
- Learning disabilities
- Obesity
- PMS
- Sensory Processing Disorder
- Tourette Syndrome
- Vision problems

A balanced glycemic diet is a grouping of foods that revolves around making choices according to the *glycemic index*, a ranking system that classifies all carbohydrates according to their effect on our blood glucose levels, and thus insulin levels. It is a quantitative measure for how rapidly 50 grams of a certain food converts to glucose or blood sugar, as it compares to 50 grams of white bread (which has a GI or glycemic index of 100).

The secret to a long, healthy life, reducing your risk of heart disease, diabetes and obesity, is to choose low and medium glycemic index carbohydrates. These are the ones that produce only small fluctuations in our blood glucose and insulin levels. They are the best for balanced brain function as well. At the same time, avoid high glycemic carbohydrates which cause glucose and insulin go haywire.

High Glycemic Index Carbohydrates – These are the foods that cause the most instability of blood sugar and metabolism. They should not be eaten on a daily basis.

- Flour Products: All white bread, all white flour products, such as pasta, cookies, pastries, cakes, pies, corn bread, most commercial cereals
- Fruits: Most dried fruits, most fruit juices, watermelon
- Grains: White rice and white rice products, corn, corn products
- Snack Foods: Potato chips, corn chips, rice cakes, pretzels
- Sweeteners: White sugar, honey, molasses, corn syrup, Sucanat, cane juice, brown sugar
- Vegetables: White potatoes, corn, turnips, parsnips

Replace instead, with the following Medium and Low Glycemic Foods:
Medium Glycemic Foods are moderate inducers of insulin. These foods are preferred to the high glycemic foods, and can be used in moderation. (Glycemic Index of 50%-80%)

- Fruits: Oranges, banana, pineapple, cantaloupe, grapes, honeydew, kiwi, mango, peaches
- Grains: Whole pumpernickel or rye bread, oatmeal (reduced cooking time), cream of buckwheat cereal, brown basmati rice, spaghetti (whole grain)
- Legumes: Black-eyed peas, navy beans, pinto beans, split peas, black beans
- Snack foods: popcorn
- Vegetables: Artichoke, peas, yams, red potatoes, carrots, beets, sweet potato

Low Glycemic Foods are the best choices.

They produce only a mild fluctuation in blood glucose and insulin levels. (Glycemic Index of 30% - 50%)

- Dairy: Whole milk, whole yogurt
- Fruits - Apple, applesauce, avocado, pears, apricot, cherries, grapefruit, lemon, lime, plums, strawberries
- Grains: Barley, buckwheat groats, oatmeal (slow cooking)
- Legumes: Lentils, kidney beans, garbanzos, lima beans, soybeans, black beans
- Sugars: Lactose, agave nectar (from cactus - similar to honey), SlimSweet (powder from kiwi), Stevia (drops or powder)
- Vegetables: Asparagus, broccoli, Brussels sprouts, cabbage, cauliflower, celery, green beans, leeks, lettuces, mushrooms, okra, onions, pea pods, peppers, radishes, spinach, sprouts, tomato, turnip greens, water chestnuts, zucchini

Note: Some foods, like nuts and seeds are not on this list because they contain very few carbohydrates. Also, animal proteins have little to no carbohydrates, so they do not cause the fluctuation in blood sugar that many carbohydrates do.

This diet can be approached very mathematically, but it is difficult to put people or food into categories or "boxes". We all have individual digestive capabilities and energy expenditures. Also, the other foods that you couple with your carbohydrates may change how glucose and insulin behave. For instance, a high fat meal with low glycemic carbohydrates may still cause an undesirable effect. That being said, using the glycemic index list as a framework for choosing food is smart. If you notice, the more natural, healthy foods are in the low and medium glycemic lists.

Glycemic Index and Glycemic Load

So, the glycemic index has its strengths and limitations because the index of a food may vary in several ways: how it is grown, how it is processed and how it is prepared. Some carbohydrates fall below others on the glycemic list but may, indeed, have a bigger impact on blood sugar. For instance, certain candy bars have a lower glycemic index than a sweet potato, but we all know who the winner is here as far as nutrient quality and healthy benefits. The sweet potato wins, hands down.[1]

To rectify the shortcomings of the glycemic index (GI), nutritionists have created the *glycemic load* (GL). It accounts for amounts and combinations of food and the impact they have on blood sugar levels. To calculate the glycemic load (GL) of a food, divide the GI by 100 and multiply by the grams of carbohydrate in the serving size.

If you don't want to fuss with "all the math", just choose foods from the low and moderate list, and think nutrient quality with your choices.

For further information and GI and GL charts, check:
www.ajcn.org/cgi/content/full/76/1/5/T1

Allergy-Free Diets

People may be allergic to one or more foods at different times in their lives and they may need to eliminate or reduce their intake. The common allergy foods for children are sugar, dairy, wheat, soy, eggs, corn, tomato, oranges, chocolate, shellfish, peanuts and tree nuts. An allergic reaction is an immune system reaction causing anything from nose, ear or throat congestion, watery eyes, to a skin rash, red cheeks, red earlobes, puffy eyes or dark circles under eyes, swollen glands, eczema, psoriasis, headaches or cravings. Focus problems, a spaced-out look, aggression, depression, stomach-aches and even flu-like symptoms may also be signs of food allergies.

Some people have delayed allergic reactions, which make the allergy foods difficult to detect. These delayed reactions often affect digestive and bowel function, emotions, behavior and sleep.

The two most useful ways of eating to halt or reduce allergic reactions are:

1. Eliminate the offending food(s) or
2. rotate foods in such a way that the body is not inundated with the same substances, day-in and day-out.

The rotation diet is explained below. Also for those people with allergies to grasses, it may be helpful to avoid eating grains (from grasses) during allergy season, especially in spring, when grass is new and pollens are plentiful.

For children who are allergic to so many foods that they have continual reactions, there is a program that supplies unusual specialty foods to you by mail. These foods are the least allergenic of any foods and have been tolerated by extremely allergic and sensitive people. You can find this program on the website: http://www.specialfoods.com.

Rotation Diet

For some people today, eating in rotation means Burger King one day, Taco Bell the next and Pizza Hut the next. But many families have implemented much stricter rotation diets as the best way to eliminate food allergies and sensitivities. You can target foods that may be culprits, those causing digestive problems, gas, bloating, stomach-aches, irritation, sinus and throat congestion, earaches, rashes, and even changes in emotions and behavior. For a more rigorous rotation diet, rotation of families of food may be necessary. Here is the basic method used to rotate foods:

1. Choose a food you think might be the cause of problems and serve it only once within 4 days. For instance, if you suspect that wheat may be an offender, then after eating wheat on Monday, don't introduce it again until Friday. This gives the body time to move it through the digestive system and adjust. Look closely for symptoms or symptom relief. Be aware that the food you intend to eliminate may be an ingredient in prepared foods, so read labels carefully. This is particularly true of corn. It helps to keep a food diary, recording symptoms accurately.
2. After reintroducing the chosen food, pay particular attention to symptoms concerning the nose, throat, ears, lungs, joints, skin, stomach and bowels. Certain behaviors may even change. If an allergic food is reintroduced, a child may become irritated, depressed or hyper. Foggy brain, tuning out and daydreaming may also be symptoms of food allergies. Challenge the body with several servings of that food.
3. Wait at least two days before eliminating the next food.
4. Experiment with any suspected allergy foods which you feel may be causing reactions.

Casein-Free Diet

Casein is a protein in cow's milk to which many people are allergic or sensitive. This is different from lactose intolerance, which is a sensitivity to lactose, the sugar in milk. A casein-free diet can be very helpful for children with allergies, asthma (even exercise-induced), autistic spectrum disorder, attention deficit disorder (ADD), attention deficit hyperactivity disorder (ADHD), celiac disease, depression, obsessive-compulsive disorder (OCD), pervasive development disorder (PDD), eczema, psoriasis, skin rashes, and many behavior and emotional imbalances.

Since casein is in cow's milk, all cow's milk products need to be eliminated: cream cheeses, cottage cheese, soft and hard cheeses, sour cream, butter, ice cream, yogurt, and milk. (See dairy alternatives that taste great and bake well in the *Healthy Substitutions Chapter 9.*) In addition to the obvious, there may be hidden casein in other foods such as bakery glazes, breath mints, coffee creamers, fortified cereals, high-protein beverage powders, infant formulas, nutrition bars, processed meats, salad dressings and whipped toppings.

Casein-containing milk products may be better tolerated by children and adults if they are eaten in their raw, whole form. Raw milk, cheese and butter contain the natural enzymes needed to digest them. These enzymes are inactivated when the dairy product is heat-treated, pasteurized and processed. Even better, homemade yogurt and kefir are alive with enzymes and beneficial bacteria, due to the fermentation process. They may be tolerated by some people with casein allergies, because in a sense, they are "pre-digested".

Another tip is to take digestive enzyme supplements, which enable more efficient breakdown of proteins, carbohydrates and fats. Since casein is a protein the body has difficulty digesting, the use of enzymes may solve the problem.

Gluten-Free Diet

(For People Who Like Interesting Food)

We rely on white flour and whole wheat products for our cereals, our sandwiches, our burgers, our "mac and cheese", our pizza, and yes, even our chicken nuggets. It is everywhere and we have created allergies to it. Over 50% of the population in North America is allergic or sensitive to wheat. You may not realize that wheat can cause constipation, diarrhea, irritable bowel syndrome, celiac disease, stomach aches, acid reflux, post-nasal drip, eczema, psoriasis, irritability, poor attention, depression and mood swings. This is because we eat too much of it. How boring. Many other grains and flours can be used which are far more interesting and a lot less allergic. Since wheat contains gluten, the first step in trying a gluten-free diet is to eliminate all whole wheat and white wheat products.

Many people with wheat or gluten allergies are already eating other grains and baking with great tasting alternative flours. Individuals with celiac disease, an auto-immune disorder, cannot eat any grains containing the sticky substance, gluten. Wheat, spelt, kamut, barley, rye and sometimes oats are off limits to them. It is for this reason that flours made from garbanzo beans, brown rice, white rice, corn, soy, potato, potato starch, tapioca, arrowroot and cassava are used. These grains and beans are dried and milled into flour that can be used in baking. From any flour, pastas, cereals, breads, cookies, cakes, muffins, pancakes and other baked goods can be made. (See C*hapter 9 on Healthy Substitutes* for specific products.)

The gluten-free grains and flours are most important for children with autistic spectrum disorder, celiac disease, gluten enteropathy, diabetes, stomach and bowel problems.[2] Children with rheumatoid arthritis, psoriasis and auto-immune thyroid disorders may benefit as well.

Some research also points to an exacerbation of symptoms in those children and teens who are manic-depressive, schizophrenic, hyperactive or bi-polar when eating gluten-containing products.[3]

Controversy surrounding "safe" and "unsafe foods" is prevalent in the gluten-free community. We have discussed this at length in *Chapters 2 and 4.* It all boils down to -- when a person eats a food to which they react poorly, they should avoid it.

"Un-Safe foods" may also apply to grains and grain products which have been contaminated with the gluten molecule. Contamination can occur:

- during preparation, with use of the common utensils or cooking surfaces
- during processing of products that go through a production line in which gluten-containing foods had preceded them
- in bulk bins which sit next to each other in the stores
- during the growing process, from neighboring fields or from other nearby plants.

Yes, some people are just that sensitive to something so specific as cross-contamination. Many people with celiac disease are reactive in this way. Because their response is called auto-immune, not a traditional **allergic response, their reactions may not occur for days,** and may be very subtle. With this condition, damage is often cumulative because a person may not feel what is happening right away.

For a full explanation of gluten-free dieting, see *Chapters 2, 4, and 9.* A word of caution: As mentioned earlier in the chapter about substitutions, gluten-free diets consisting of high amounts of rice, potato, soy and tapioca flours can be disruptive to a child's blood sugar balance. This can lead to hypoglycemia, diabetes, obesity, poor focus and concentration, and mood disorders. Many gluten-free flour products are refined and should be used cautiously, as treats.

The following websites offer a wide selection of gluten-free products:

www.ener-g.com
www.glutenfree-foods.co.uk
www.glutenfree.com
www.wholefoodsmarket.com

The GF/CF or Gluten-Free/Casein-Free Diet

The GF/CF diet is a gluten-free, casein-free diet. Avoidance of both gluten and casein may be helpful for more people than you might imagine. Certainly, children with autistic spectrum disorder, celiac disease, and gluten and casein allergies benefit from the diet. I educate all my patients about the importance of avoiding, or at least rotating, gluten and casein, whether they have a diagnosis or not.

It makes so much sense to minimize the intake of products with these two molecules, as they dominate the food industry and we can become saturated with them. Nature has given us a wide variety of food and we should take advantage of that. (See *Substitutions Chapter 9*)

For those with autistic spectrum disorder, gluten and casein may be extremely harmful, due to possible leakage of these proteins from the gut into the bloodstream. This may cause the body's immune system to attack the foreign proteins, creating inflammatory reactions and activating the opiate receptors of the brain. In other words, some autistic children might even appear to be "drugged" and react emotionally and behaviorally unusual. Intense cravings for gluten and casein-containing foods are very common and may appear to be like addictions. A person may act as if they can't live in that moment without a particular food. They will want only these foods and no others.

A three-month trial without gluten and casein foods would give enough time to see if there is any behavioral improvement. For many, the diet should be continued indefinitely. Up to 8 in 10 autistic children exhibit improved socialization, concentration, learning, verbalization, among many other behavioral improvements after sustaining a 100% gluten-free, casein-free diet.

Ketogenic Diet

The ketogenic diet has been used since the 1920s in the treatment of epilepsy. The diet is a restricted calorie diet, high in fat and low in carbohydrates and protein. This results in a change in body chemistry called ketosis. In the state of ketosis, the body is tricked into burning fat instead of glucose for energy, causing a semi-fasting condition. An anti-epileptic effect is then exerted. Fluids are also limited, which helps contribute to the diet's success. The ketogenic diet seems to work best for ages 1-10; two out of three children are able to eliminate or reduce the frequency of their seizures. Some teens and adults have success when they use the diet, but the statistics are much lower.

You must consult with a knowledgeable health professional when using the ketogenic diet. Choosing the right foods and weighing them, contribute to the success of this program. Fatty foods, cream, dips and unheated oils are utilized along with some fish and animal proteins, as well as carefully chosen carbohydrates. The diet has a 4 to 1 ratio of fat to protein and carbohydrates.

Blood and urine tests are routinely done by your doctor, as the diet does have side effects. It is dehydrating and can cause problems with the kidneys and liver. A study in the August 2000 issue of the Journal of Urology indicates that some children with refractory epilepsy develop kidney stones when on the ketogenic diet after about eighteen months.[4]

Although often successful in preventing seizures, continued use of this diet, more than 18 months is not advised. Other side effects may be high fats in the blood, gallstones, acidosis, dehydration, slow growth rate, lethargy and constipation.

It is very important to give the child appropriate vitamin and mineral supplementation when they are on the ketogenic diet, as it only offers about 75% of the Recommended Daily Allowances (RDAs) for vitamins and minerals. Digestive enzyme capsules put in the food or taken as a supplement may also be helpful for enhancing digestion and absorption of concentrated protein and fat-containing foods.

Feingold Program and Diet

The work of the Feingold Association to increase awareness of the harmful effects of food and synthetic additives is commendable. A non-profit organization, they disseminate information about how to avoid and replace these foods, as well as the role they play in the treatment of behavior, learning and health problems.

The program is based on a diet eliminating synthetic colors, synthetic flavors and the preservatives BHA, BHT and TBHQ. This elimination diet is composed of 2 stages:

Stage One: The initial period requires that you remove from your diet, the items listed below in order to obtain a favorable response. Many of these items are phenol-based, derived from petroleum.

- BHA (Butylated Hydroxyanisole)
- BHT (Butylated Hydroxytoluene)
- Natural Salicylates
- Synthetic (Artificial) Colors
- Synthetic (Artificial) Flavors
- TBHQ (Tertiary Butylhydroquinone)

The following foods contain naturally-occurring salicylates and should be avoided in any form, whether garden-fresh, canned, dried, frozen or juiced.

- Almonds
- Apples
- Apricots
- Berries (all)
- Cherries
- Chili powder
- Cider and cider vinegar
- Cloves
- Coffee, tea
- Cucumbers and pickles
- Currants
- Grapes and raisins
- Nectarines, peaches
- Oil of wintergreen (methyl salicylate)
- Oranges
- Paprika
- Peppers (bell and chili)
- Plums and prunes

- Tangerines
- Tomatoes
- Wine and wine vinegar

Aspirin and medication containing aspirin should also be avoided.

Stage Two: Try Stage Two if you have a good response to Stage One for four to six weeks. Reintroduce the natural salicylate items above, very carefully, one at a time, every few days, watching for reactions. The Feingold Association offers a handbook, *Once You See Improvement*, to help you implement this stage.

When you become a member, you receive a handbook, food lists, recipes, menu plans, product alerts, a medication guide and a newsletter. This collection is not to be surpassed in its thoroughness and simplicity. Find out more by visiting their website at www.feingold.org or calling 800-321-3287.

Many children and adults with behavior, learning and health problems have been helped with this program.[5] Actually everyone could benefit by following the basic Feingold Program, eliminating chemical preservatives, additives and colorings. It is sound advice for the human body.

The PAMM Diet

Pan-Asian Modified Mediterranean Diet

More and more children are being diagnosed with high blood pressure and hypertension, due to being overweight or obese. Blood pressure can be normalized without medications in as little as eight weeks. The answer is right in your refrigerator.[6]

The PAMM Diet combines all natural, fresh foods from the Mediterranean areas of Italy, Greece and Spain with foods from the Asian cuisine. The diet also recommends walking 1-2 miles daily to reach your goal.

The typical Mediterranean diet includes lots of fresh fruit and vegetables, local fish, olive oil, fresh garlic and nuts to lower blood pressure and cholesterol levels. The Asian diet is bountiful in fish, fresh vegetables and fruits, locally-harvested seaweeds and soy products, and offers many of the same benefits.

Specifically, fish are an important part of the PAMM Diet because they are rich in omega-3 fatty acids and coenzyme Q10 to reduce inflammation, blood pressure and excessive blood clotting. Nuts, seeds, garlic and olive oil also have similar benefits.

Finally, the PAMM Diet is rich in the low-glycemic foods that are so important for blood sugar stabilization. Lentils, garbanzo beans, soybeans and other legumes provide plant protein plus low-glycemic carbohydrates. Saturated fats are reduced with a focus on olive oil consumption, so the diet promotes healthy arteries, better blood flow and balanced weight.

Admittedly, it may be difficult to keep children on this diet. A good idea is to have the whole family commit to a structure like this for two months, in order to reach an important health goal. Once blood pressures and cholesterol levels have normalized, you can then vary your food intake, using the PAMM foods as a framework.

Vegetarianism and Children

There is a growing group of young vegetarians. However, if your child announces that he or she is never going to eat meat again, they may or may not mean it. When some children make the connection between eating flesh and the animals they love, it can cause them to shift their taste buds toward non-meat foods. This may last for a few days -- maybe longer. With growing interest in the environment among young people today, vegetarianism has returned as a popular trend. Unfortunately, the transition to vegetarianism is not often accompanied by a newfound craving for quinoa, black beans, sunflower seeds or greens.[7]

Kids are kids. Vegetarian children often turn to a high carbohydrate diet and junk foods when they eliminate the flesh foods. Parents may feel lost about providing the right kinds of food for their veggie children, but the health food industry has taken care of that. There is a world of vegetarian options, now more than ever, that appeal to young children and teens. Most kids love bean burritos, veggie sub sandwiches, tofu hot dogs, and vegetarian pizza.

Children, especially teens, may think that as long as they don't eat any animals, they are eating healthfully. But they share a common set of nutritional requirements with their meat-eating peers. A balanced and nourishing vegetarian diet <u>can</u> be achieved according to the American Dietetic Association. Both vegans eating no animal products, and lacto-ovo vegetarians eating dairy and eggs, are appropriate for all stages of the life cycle, including young children and teens. However, it is important to pay attention to the following nutrients:

Vitamin B-12: 2.5 to 3 mcg daily is important for brain function, digestion and blood cell production. Vegetarian sources include tempeh, sea vegetables, blue green algae, nutritional yeast, yogurt and tofu. With enough friendly intestinal bacteria, the body can manufacture B-12. Therefore, taking acidophilus and bifidus supplements is advised.

Protein: Kids require between 30-40 grams of protein daily to insure proper tissue growth and repair, brain neurotransmission and the manufacture of hormones. Essential amino acids which are the building blocks of protein are contained in dairy products, eggs, legumes, seeds, whey protein powder, tofu, soy foods and algae products. Combining together such foods as grains and legumes can make up for certain amino acid deficiencies in single foods.

Calcium is necessary for the growth of bones and teeth, as well as the brain and nervous system. Children should obtain 800-1,000 mg. daily from such plant sources as: soybeans, other legumes, tofu, soymilk, seeds, almonds, dark leafy greens and broccoli.

Vitamin D is essential for calcium absorption and utilization. Sun exposure for 5-15 minutes every day may provide enough, and supplements are also available.

Iron (10-15 mg.) is needed daily by children for blood building and brain function. Research has linked iron deficiency to anemia and impaired learning and memory in students. Vegetarian sources include seeds, legumes, nuts, spinach, tomato, eggs, and whole or fortified grain products.

Zinc is important for growth, immune function and many aspects of brain function. It is plentiful in grains, bran and other cereals, pumpkin seeds, legumes and many vegetables, but is lost in the processing of these foods, so make sure your vegetarian child consumes the unprocessed versions.

Essential fatty acids, especially omega 3's, are important for cardiovascular health, brain development and brain function. Deficiencies have been tied to depression, learning and behavioral disorders, asthma, allergies and skin problems. Plant sources include flax, hemp and pumpkin seeds and their oils. Most nuts, especially walnuts and seeds are good sources of essential fatty acids and healthiest when eaten raw.

Soy products are popular for vegetarian children. Highly processed soy products such as isolates and powders may appear to be good protein sources, but are poorly digested and can cause gas and bloating. This may lead to intestinal and bowel problems, as well as allergies. Because soy contains a high amount of plant estrogens, eating too much may also disrupt a child's hormone imbalance. When consuming soy products, children should be encouraged to use miso, tofu, natto (fermented soybeans), and tempeh, as these are closest to the original source. Most of these foods are fermented and are, therefore, better digested.

Diet for ADD and ADHD Children and Adults

Numerous studies in peer-reviewed journals discuss the diagnosis and treatment of ADD and ADHD in children. In one such study, the American Academy of Pediatrics issues guidelines to help physicians diagnose these conditions. Mention is made that they are currently developing recommendations for treatment. These treatment options are either drug or behaviorally-oriented.[8]

I say why bother? Why spend millions of dollars on research when we already have the answers. Parents, naturopaths, nutritionists, acupuncturists, chiropractors and other natural practitioners are already having success with ADD/ADHD. Let's wake up and address the allergies, the blood sugar imbalances, the toxic overload and the digestive problems.

When these physical imbalances are addressed through the use of whole foods, superfoods and nutritional supplementation, the ADHD symptoms often reduce or disappear. This is one of the reasons I wrote this book - so people can access information that they are not getting in the doctor's office or from the schools. Foods heal - if you choose the right ones.

My recommendations for children and adults with the ADD or ADHD diagnosis are the allergy-free diet, GF/CF diet, the Feingold Diet and balanced glycemic diet.

---

1. *www.ajcn.org*
2. *"Gluten-Free Diet Early in Life May Prevent Autoimmune Diseases in Celiac Patients," Journal of Pediatrics, August 2000; 137: pp.263-265.*
3. *Philpott, William H, M.D. and Kalita, Dwight K, Ph.D, Brain Allergies: The Psychonutrient Connection, Keats Publishing, Inc, 1980.*
4. *Kielb, S, M.D., et al, "Ketogenic Diet Linked With High Rate of Kidney Stones," Journal of Urology, August 2000; 164: pp.464-466.*
5. *Hersey, J, Why Can't My Child Behave?, Pear Tree Press, 1999.*
6. *"You Can Lower Your Blood Pressure in Eight Weeks", Sinatra, S, MD, www.drsinatra.com*
7. *"Wanted: Veggie Options with Kid Appeal", Keeler, B, Thompson, LN, Ph.D., Natural Foods Merchandiser.*
8. *American Academy of Pediatrics, "Clinical practice guideline: diagnosis and evaluation of the child with attention-deficit/hyperactivity disorder," Journal of Pediatrics, 2000; 105: pp.1158-1170.*

Chapter Twelve

A PLAN FOR WINNING: Sports Nutrition for Kids

Studying Physical "Un-Fitness"

The more I observe the world of youngsters today, the more I reflect on my very physically active childhood. I won't bore you with the details – I'm sure you have similar memories. Look around you now. Have you ever seen so many out-of-shape children and teens?

On the other hand, many kids today are incredibly active but their schedules are more structured, less spontaneous than in "yesteryears". Other children are extremely sedentary, addicted to TV, computers and video games. On the positive side, I'm sure something good can come from computer and video game activities – persistence and mental fortitude, to start with.

But all in all, when you sit on your butt for hours "on end", blood, oxygen and nutrients do not circulate to the muscles, joints and bones, the way they would if you were running a race or jumping in the leaves. Add poor quality meals and snack foods to that equation, and you get physically un-fit children. The health implications down the road may be devastating. Let's look at some facts:

Youth at Risk: One in Three Kids Not Physically Fit
Journal of the American Medical Association, December 21, 2005; 294(23): 2981-2988

More than a third of U.S. adolescents are physically unfit. They are at greater risk of developing heart disease as they age. Over 3,000 adolescents were asked to walk or run on a treadmill, after which their heart and blood pressure were measured. About 34 percent were at the lowest possible fitness level. This could mean up to 7.5 million adolescents, ages 12 to 19 nationwide are unfit. The unfit teens were also twice as likely to be overweight, and two to three times as likely to have high cholesterol.

Physical Inactivity & Poor Diet Lead to Obesity & Fatigue in Children
"The 'skinny' on childhood obesity: how our western environment starves kids' brains." Lustig RH, Pediatric Annals 35:12, December 2006, 898-907

In this review, the author details certain causes of obesity in children: He suggests:

- Exercise by playing, bike riding, playing sports & walking 30 minutes daily.
- Stop buying sweets and soda. Use the substitution list for better choices.
- Have your children help you prepare meals. Make a game of it.
- Limit TV time to help with the addiction of tuning out and being lazy.
- Plan activities -- a trip to the library, playground or park. Keep moving.

"U.S. children's blood pressure rising: increases found among kids of all ages, racial groups", Muntner, Paul of Tulane University, New Orleans, Journal of the American Medical Association, May 5, 2004

Blood-pressure levels are rising among young Americans, raising concern over potential health problems when the children grow up. The study suggests that what children eat and how much they exercise may be important factors -- in addition to previously recognized weight problems -- contributing to the increase.
"These results suggest that in another 10 to 20 years we will be facing much higher rates of hypertension, heart disease and stroke as these children become adults."

Sedentary Behavior Diminishes Lung Function
"The Increase of Childhood Chronic Conditions in the US", James M. Perrin, MD; Sheila R. Bloom, MS; Steven L. Gortmaker, PhD, Journal of American Medical Association, 2007;297:2755-2759.

Excerpt from study: An association between asthma and obesity supports the theory that sedentary behavior diminishes lung function, researchers said. With more time indoors, children also have increased exposure to indoor allergens.

"Alzheimer's Dementia Linked to Idleness During Youth"
From the London Times, March 5, 2001 (United Press International)

In this study, led by scientist, Robert Friedman at University Hospitals of Cleveland in Ohio, diversity and intensity of recreational, physical and intellectual activities were reduced in the people who went on to develop Alzheimer's. Participants in the study had, overall, 26 different activities, including: football, swimming, gardening, watching television and roller-skating.

The Tide Is Turning

There is a tremendous focus on organized sports in the world of today's family. There is no state or federal law requiring that physical education be provided in the U.S. public school system. There are, however, national recommendations:

National Recommendations:

- School-age youth should participate daily in 60 minutes or more of moderate to vigorous physical activity that is developmentally appropriate, enjoyable, and involves a variety of activities.[1,2,3]
- All elementary school students should participate in physical education for at least 150 minutes per week. All middle and high school students should participate for at least 225 minutes per week. [4,5,6,7,8,]

Sadly, many children are not meeting these recommendations. Study after report after census indicates that children are getting less regular physical activity than ever. The repercussions of this, health-wise, are serious. We are only, now, beginning to see the effects: more obesity, higher risk of cardiovascular disease, higher cholesterol and triglyceride blood levels.

Participation in Physical Activity by Young People

Grunbaum, J. A., Kann, L., Kinchen, S., Ross, J., Hawkins, J., Lowry, R., Harris, W. A., et al. (2004). Youth risk behavior surveillance—United States, 2003. Morbidity and Mortality Weekly Report, 53(SS-2), 1-95.

-- Over a third of 9th-12th graders do not engage in regular, vigorous physical activity.
-- One-third of 9th-12th graders do not engage in sufficient moderate to vigorous physical activity.
-- Over 11 percent of 9th-12th graders get no moderate to vigorous physical activity.
-- As children get older, participation in physical activity decreases. 69 percent of ninth graders and 55 percent of 12th graders participate in vigorous regular physical activity.
-- Overall, among high school students, males are more physically active than females and white students are more active than black and Hispanic students.

So, we have a double whammy: 1) children are sedentary, with of lots of stimulus that requires sitting, 2) physical education has been cut back in many school systems and eliminated in others.

How do parents weigh-in on this? More than 75 percent of parents, as well as teachers believe that school boards should not eliminate phys-ed classes for budgetary reasons or the need to meet stricter academic standards. But, this is what's happening.[9]

And, the burden of responsibility goes to 1) the parent, to ensure the child engages in physical activity, 2) the teacher, to deal with antsy students and 3) the community or private organizations, to offer organized sports activities. That is, indeed, what is happening.

Even if physical education cuts have affected your school, student physical activity levels can be increased through elementary school recess, physical activity breaks, physical activity clubs, special events and good, old-fashioned playing outside.

Positive Results for Active Kids

Playing and exercise are important for children of all ages. They enhance bone growth, circulation, metabolism and brain cell function. **Bike riding, swimming and athletic activities should be at least 30 minutes to one hour daily.** This is more important now than ever, since up to 80% of the physical education classes in the public schools in the U.S. have been cut.

Brain Cells Double with Exercise

"New neurons in old brains: learning to survive?" Greenough WT, Cohen NJ, Juraska JM, Nature Neuroscience, March 1999, 2:203 – 205

A fascinating study in Nature Neuroscience revealed that rats that ran on an exercise wheel "whenever they wanted" had the ability to grow two times as many brain cells in the region of the hippocampus (part of the brain involved in memory and learning) than those who did not have exercise wheels in their cages.

Physical activity has also been found to help with balanced moods and emotions. The following study suggests that incorporating regular physical activity into children's lives may be a "low-risk" alternative to drug treatment.

"Active Kids Less Prone to Depression"

Motl, Robert. Psychosomatic Medicine, May-June 2004; vol 66: pp 336-342

In a study of nearly 4,600 middle-schoolers followed for two years, researchers found that the more active children were, the less likely they were to be depressed.

According to Dr. Rod Dishman (University of Georgia), "Exercise could plausibly help prevent depression ... as well as treat it. The benefits of exercise generally take longer to emerge compared with drug treatment. With adolescents, the safety of drug treatment is not certain, and since psychological therapy is not always effective, it is important to keep studying "low-risk" alternatives, such as physical activity.

Positive effects of exercise on dietary habits and health have also been documented. The study below also indicates that physically active children and adolescents have better eating habits and are, thus, healthier than those who are less active. This is no surprise, but it's good to see the science behind the logic.

"Children Who Play Sports Have Better Eating Habits",
Kroll, JK, et al, Journal of the American Dietetic Association, May 2006; 106:709-717.

Adolescents involved in weight-related and power team sports have better eating habits and nutrient intake than their non-sports involved peers, say researchers at University of Minnesota. Nutrient demands increase when playing sports.

Over 4,700 junior high and high school students were studied for their meal and snack frequency, energy and nutrient intake and physical activity. Researchers found "sport-involved youth generally ate breakfast more frequently and had higher lean protein, calcium, iron and zinc intakes than their non-sport involved peers. These findings support a positive association between adolescent sports participation and health."

All in all, it makes so much sense, that when the brain's fuel – oxygen and glucose – is circulating more with exercise of some type, a person, a child will have multiple benefits. Below is just one of the many studies that summarize those benefits:

Benefits of Physical Activity
Dwyer, T., Sallis, J. F., Blizzard, L., Lazarus, R., & Dean, K. (2001). Relation of Academic Performance to Physical Activity and Fitness in Children. Pediatric Exercise Science, 13, 225-238.

Youth receiving additional physical activity tend to show improved attributes such as:
-- increased brain function and nourishment

-- higher energy and concentration levels
-- positive changes in body build, affecting self esteem
-- increased self-esteem and better behavior, which may all support cognitive learning.

Adults benefit from exercise in much the same way that children do. This is why smart business leaders and CEO's of major corporations have treadmills in their offices – for clearer decision-making, better memory and focus.[10]

Where to Exercise Caution

Growing bodies are vulnerable to injury and imbalance. Research about participants in weight-related sports such as wrestling, gymnastics and weight lifting indicates that energy and nutrient intakes of calcium, iron, zinc and vitamin D may be below recommended levels in some athletes[11] Certain studies also indicate that wrestlers, gymnasts, figure skaters and those focused on their weight and body image, may develop dysfunctional eating patterns. I can remember the wrestlers in my high school inducing vomiting and taking laxatives in order to "make weight". Other studies have shown that female athletes are more prone to development of eating disorders.[12]

We think of exercise and sports as activities that build the body, condition the body. They do, but they also cause a certain amount of catabolic activity that "tears down" muscle and other tissues. This is part of the process. A problem occurs, however, when the athlete does not take in or eat the nutrients that build and repair the body's tissues. The bones, muscles, tendons and ligaments will suffer. Add insult to injury when the athlete uses foods and beverages that cause more tearing down, such as in the following example:

"Teenaged Girls, Carbonated Beverage Consumption and Bone Fractures"
Wyshak, Grace, PhD, Archives of Pediatric Adolescent Med. 2000; 154:610-613.

The study with 9th and 10th grade girls in an urban high school, confirmed that cola drinks are associated with more bone fractures in physically active girls.

Comment: This was one of the studies that caused national concern and alarm about the health impact of carbonated beverage consumption and led to the movement still happening today – which restricts carbonated beverages from vending machines in the schools of some towns and states.

The following nutritional problems may occur in some athletes or highly active children:

1. **Excess calcium loss** - Taking the above study a step further – excessive cola and soda consumption can lead to calcium loss. This, of course, affects not only bones, but all tissues in the body. For instance, calcium is also important for calming the nervous system. Teenage girls who do intense weight training can have premature bone loss. They are advised to take about 600 mg. of calcium citrate daily with 300 mg. of magnesium, and eliminate soda consumption. This holds true for boys too. In fact, we've seen a higher incidence of injuries among young athletes in the last ten years, due to poor calcium and mineral intake, as well as calcium loss from ingesting carbonated beverages.
2. **Iron loss** - Athletes who work out rigorously use their stores of iron more quickly than non-athletes -- especially menstruating girls, but boys too. This can damage the neurological system, as well as weaken the blood cells. Use iron-rich foods: leafy greens, beets, berries and legumes. Also, certain whey proteins enhance iron absorption.
3. **Electrolyte loss** - Sweaty workouts and athletic events cause people to lose electrolytes -- potassium, magnesium and sodium through perspiration and urination. These minerals are responsible for regulating body water, muscle contraction and heart rhythms. It is important to use an electrolyte replacement drink after physical activity. A better choice than Gatorade is Recharge, available in several flavors. Another is Emergen-C, made by Alacer. All are available in the health food stores. Your health care practitioner may have specific products they recommend. I recommend Rehydration and Spectra Min drops by Energetix, added to water or another beverage.
4. **Excess intake of caffeine** – Repetitive use of energy and sports drinks containing caffeine can cause "Toxic Jock Syndrome". This is explained as an increased tendency to risky behavior and aggression due to excessive use of caffeine.
5. **Caution with antibiotics** - Be careful if a child or teen is taking or has just taken antibiotics. Certain antibiotics have been found to weaken the tendons of the knees, calves, thighs and shoulders, making people more susceptible to injury. Weight training, high-impact or strenuous athletic activities should be performed with caution at this time.

Problems with or Extreme Sports & Over-Scheduling

Millions of children across North America feel overwhelmed. Parents today feel they are not being good parents if they don't give their children everything they never had. So, the new parenting motive is to fit it ALL in - ballet, baseball, swimming, football, tennis and the next play date. Be aware of the problems which may result from stressful over-scheduling. Example: A 4am wakeup call to practice swimming for 2 hours before school can disrupt the circadian rhythm of the body and cause hormonal imbalances: fatigue, mood swings, depression, anxiety, sleep problems, poor appetite and weight gain or loss. Balance is the key here.

What happens to a child when there are intense training schedules and the ever- present pressure to win and to be #1? The answer is ... physical burnout, mental exhaustion, chronic fatigue and injuries. Would it be shocking to know this is happening as early as age 9 or 10?

Kids' sports have become much more competitive," says Dr. Jordan Metzl, Medical Director of the Sports Medicine Institute for Young Athletes at the Hospital for Special Surgery in New York City. "And in general, high-level competition for young kids is not a great thing," says Metzl, co-author of *"The Young Athlete: A Sports Doctor's Complete Guide for Parents."*[13]

With more kids than ever in organized sports, an estimated 30 million of them up through high school, Metzl and other experts in sports medicine and youth athletics say they are increasingly concerned about the pressures put on some children to excel. Not only are these youngsters at risk for emotional burnout, they may also develop injuries that plague them for a lifetime. Some will turn to steroids or other performance-enhancing substances to try to gain an edge. And some may give up on sports -- and exercise – altogether, because, after all, where's the fun in it?

More and more teenagers, athletes and non-athletes are turning to anabolic steroids. In the United States, about 3 million people use anabolic steroids — one in four of these steroid users started as a teenager, and one out of every 10 <u>is</u> a teenager.[14]

Anabolic means muscle-building and steroids are synthetic substances, similar to the male hormone, testosterone. Growth hormone is also a steroid. Anabolic steroids come in tablets, injections, patches and gels. Doctors prescribe a different kind of steroid, called corticosteroids, to reduce swelling and inflammation. Corticosteroids are not anabolic steroids and do not have the same harmful effects. But doctors don't prescribe anabolic steroids to young, healthy people to help them build muscles. Without a prescription from a doctor, steroids are illegal.

Young athletes are looking for leaner, more muscular bodies, with more speed, strength and endurance. Most teenage steroid-users are entranced by athletes and movie stars and want to enhance their self image. There is tremendous secrecy around this topic. While some teens hide their use by calling the steroids – supplements, others deny it altogether. But the fact remains that thousands of teenage boys and girls, over a quarter of a million, eighth through twelfth grades, have used steroids, according to a survey by the University of Michigan's Institute for Social Research. The survey shows that steroid use is on the rise and that teens are getting them from friends, drug dealers and older athletes. Indications are that steroid use is the highest among senior boys and athletes.[15]

Steroid Use Among Teenage Boys

Monitoring the Future: National Results on Adolescent Drug Use, Overview of Key Findings, Johnston, LD, PhD, et al, 2006, p. 43 (U.S. Department of Health and Human Services, National Institutes of Health)

2.7% of high school seniors use steroids. Anabolic steroids can halt bone growth and result in a permanently short stature, so they're particularly dangerous for still-growing adolescents. Steroids can also damage the heart and liver.

Steroid use with teenage girls is on the rise and it is not only reserved for the athletes, as the study below indicates.

"Cross-sectional Study: Female Students Report Anabolic Steroid Use",

Elliot, DL, MD; Cheong, J, PhD; Moe, EL, PhD, MPH; Goldberg, L, MD, Arch Pediatr Adolesc Med. June 2007;161:572-577

A national survey of high schools showed that 5.3 percent of teen girls admitted to using or having used anabolic steroids, which are synthetic substances related to male sex hormones and are illegal without a prescription. The girls, including cheerleaders and non-athletic girls, used steroids to enhance their self image.

Anabolic steroids can also lead to early heart attacks, strokes, liver tumors, kidney failure and serious psychiatric problems. Eventually, steroids can cause mania, delusions, and violent aggression or "roid rage." Signs your son may be taking anabolic steroids include increased acne and male-pattern baldness. If your daughter takes anabolic steroids, she may develop male characteristics, such as a deep voice or dark facial hair. Educate yourselves and your children about the hazardous effects of performance-enhancing drugs. Encourage your children to build from the foundation-up or from the inside-out. The next section will empower you to use "foundation-up" nutrition to its fullest.

Super Nutrition for Pre-Game or Activity

How to enhance energy, strength, endurance and focus

1. For pre-workout, performance or a game, eat a large meal with complex carbohydrates at least 3-4 hours beforehand or a small meal 2 hours before.
2. Always use digestive enzymes with the meal to enhance proper digestion and absorption of nutrients and support muscle energy.
3. Carbohydrate-loading several days before an athletic event produces better results for endurance, but not speed. Complex carbohydrates like oatmeal, brown rice, vegetables and legumes (for instance, a black bean burrito) are better choices than pizza, pasta or sugar foods. And ... they produce better results.
4. Support adrenal glands with B vitamins, including B5, B6, along with minerals, zinc and chromium.
5. Zinc aids in tissue repair and adrenal function.
6. Vitamin E and selenium are important antioxidants, especially for aerobic athletes. Aerobic exercise increases free radical damage and cellular damage, but that is lessened with vitamin E and selenium. They also improve immune function. (Vitamin E = 400 IU, selenium = 200 mcg. for kids over 120 pounds)
7. The amino acid, glutamine, can be low after prolonged exercise. This can deplete the white blood cell count, impairing immune function and causing more susceptibility to colds, flues and allergies. Glutamine can be taken in capsule or powder form. It also helps repair and build muscle.
8. For endurance and to build your energy "storehouse":
9. Eat a complex carbohydrate and protein post activity, such as oatmeal or quinoa hot cereal. Stir in some whey and goat or rice milk. A combo like this helps move insulin from the bloodstream to the muscles for energy.
10. Consider using an amino acid supplement with arganine and ornithine, or use capsules of blue green algae, a good source amino acids.

Sometimes Misunderstood

Protein is not an energy food; it builds and repairs muscles. High protein, low carbohydrate diets don't work for all athletes. Body builders function better on them than runners or those playing competitive games. This is because high protein diets can be very dehydrating and runners, as well as other competitive athletes, can become dehydrated more quickly than body builders. This can lead to weak muscles, foggy brain and fatigue.

Fat-free or low-fat diets do not enhance athletic performance. It is important to eat the good fats – avocado, nuts, seeds -- and at the right time, not immediately following a workout. Fats are a source of energy and fuel, so fatigue and emotional imbalances can develop from eating a low-fat diet. Healthy fats also help build hormones and low-fat diets can also cause adrenal, thyroid or sex hormone imbalances. Poor mental focus and concentration may also result.

Recovery Nutrition

Athletes who work out for 60 minutes or more in high, intense situations should pay particular attention to nourishing the body properly within 15-30 minutes after the activity. This is the window of time when the muscles act "like a sponge", soaking up the food you eat. Complex carbohydrates and protein are the foods of choice.

- Avoid too much protein post activity, as this can cause the production of cholecystokinin or CCK, which hinders the rate of absorption of food into the intestines and the rate of recovery. Some experts recommend a 4:1 rate of carbohydrates to protein at this time.
- Eat very little fat post workout or game. Fat at this time slows down absorption of food through the intestines.

The following areas are of interest for recovery from physical activity:

- Electrolyte and mineral balance – ionized minerals and electrolyte drink help replenish the body's tissues after high activity and sweating
- Bone support – calcium, magnesium, boron and vitamin D help feed the bones
- Ligament and muscle support – minerals, such as magnesium and potassium, help control muscle spasms and alleviate cramping. Amino acids help to repair damaged tissue.
- Toxin elimination – use antioxidant foods and supplement to neutralize the free radicals created by exercise and catabolic activity
- Inflammation protection – proteolytic enzymes, such as protease, and amino acids, like glutamine help reduce inflammation
- Tissue healing – topical creams and gels with arnica, MSM, amino acids, and essential oils are good for healing from injuries. Oxicell (by Apex Energetics) is a glutathione cream helps relieve pain and inflammation.

Supplements & Nutrients That Enhance Athletic Performance

1. **Protein powders** – Whey, rice and hemp are better choices than soy, as soy is highly processed and can be highly allergenic.
2. **Amino acid supplements** – Amino acid capsules or powder may enhance muscle strength and better mental focus. Blue green algae is a

natural food supplement, containing many essential and non-essential amino acids.

3. **Gamma oryzanol**, derived from rice bran oil, is used to increase muscle mass and strength and reduce body fat.
4. **B-complex vitamins** are vital for energy production, mental focus and concentration, as well as recovery from the stress of intense physical activity.
5. **Co-Q-10** supplies oxygen to the muscles. It is vital for producing cellular energy.
6. **Creatine**, a naturally-occurring compound in animal tissue, is used in pill or powder form by athletes to increase ATP formation and enhance muscular endurance. It is controversial, since there are no long-term studies on it.
7. **Chromium picolinate** enhances fat burning and increases muscle mass.
8. **Essential fatty acids** from cod liver oil, tuna, wild salmon, blue green algae, nuts, seeds and lecithin provide the building blocks to hormones, and are essential for collagen formation as well as joint flexibility.
9. **Glucosamine sulfate** is a natural substance critical for the joint tissue. It enhances joint repair by stimulating the synthesis of collagen. Because of this, it has the effect of relieving pain and inflammation with no side effects. It has been found in several studies to surpass Ibuprofen in the relief of pain. It is also protective against joint destruction.
10. **Magnesium** is a mineral that is vital for energy production and muscle support. It helps with flexibility, cramps, pain relief and ligament and tendon strength.
11. **MSM** (Methosulfonylmethane) is a rich natural form of sulfur, a fundamental mineral. It is essential in the formation of skin, connective tissue and cartilage. It is found in formulas to enhance recovery, as it has anti-inflammatory and pain-reducing properties.
12. **Brain foods** - New trends in sports nutrition are to energize the brain by supporting alertness, concentration and focus. If you support brain function you can exercise longer, with more ease. Many athletes report better focus and concentration, improving the quality of their performance with specific brain foods such as: deep-sea fish, eggs, whey protein, avocado, almonds, sunflower seeds, lecithin, flax seed oil, rice bran oil, cod liver oil and blue green algae.

Tips for Enhancing the Benefits of Physical Activity

- Remember to stretch and cool down. Children and teens should be guided to allow their bodies to recoup and rebuild after long practices, games or competitions. All athletes do this.
- Make sure that your child takes part in physical activity requiring hand-eye coordination. Experts agree that these types of activities are essential to a child's development.
- To obtain optimal mental and physical energy, your child should eat 5 small meals daily or 3 regular meals interspersed with 2 healthy snacks. (See *Chapter 10 on Easy Meals.*)
- If your child is not interested in team sports, encourage him or her to engage in martial arts, yoga, Qi-gong or other individual physical activities.
- Some children are not attracted to sports of any type. Encourage them to stretch, walk, jump rope or do calisthenics. You can make it a family activity. The brain benefits from regular circulation of oxygen and glucose. Your kids will too.

---

1. *Strong, W. B., Malina, R. M., Bumkie, C. J. R., Daniels, S. R., Dishman, R. K., Gutin, B., Hergenroeder, A. C., Must, A., Nixon, P. A., Pivarnik, J. M., Rowland, T., Trost, S., & Trudeau, F. (2005). Evidence based physical activity for school-age youth. Journal of Pediatrics, 146, 732-737.*
2. *U.S. Department of Agriculture & U.S. Department of Health and Human Services. (2000). Nutrition and your health: Dietary guidelines for Americans (5th ed.). Washington, DC: Author.*
3. *National Association for Sport and Physical Education. (2004). Physical activity for children: A statement of guidelines for children ages 5-12 (2nd ed.). Reston, VA: Author.*
4. *National Association for Sport and Physical Education. (2000). Opportunity to learn standards for elementary school physical education. Reston, VA: Author.*
5. *National Association for Sport and Physical Education. (2004). Opportunity to learn standards for middle school physical education. Reston, VA: Author.*
6. *National Association for Sport and Physical Education. (2004). Opportunity to learn standards for high school physical education. Reston, VA: Author.*
7. *National Association of State Boards of Education. (2000). Fit, healthy, and ready to learn: A school health policy guide. Part 1: Physical activity, healthy eating, and tobacco-use prevention. Alexandria, VA: Author.*
8. *Centers for Disease Control and Prevention. (1997). Guidelines for school and community programs to promote lifelong physical activity among young people. Morbidity and Mortality Weekly Report, 46(No.RR-6), 1-36.*

9. *Robert Wood Johnson Foundation. (2003). National poll shows parents and teachers agree on solutions to childhood obesity [News release]. Princeton, NJ*
10. *Medina, J, Brain Rules: 12 Principles for Surviving & Thriving at Work, Home, School, Pear Press, Seattle, WA, 2008.*
11. *Thompson, JL, Energy balance in young athletes. Int Journal of Sports Nutrition, 1998; 8:160-174.*
12. *Golden, NH, A review of the female athlete triad (amenorrhea, osteoporosis and disordered eating), Int Journal of Adolescent Medical Health, 2002; 14:9-17.*
13. *The Young Athlete: A Sports Doctor's Complete Guide for Parents, Metzl JD, MD and Shookhoff, Carol, April 2003, Little, Brown and Company.*
14. *Mayo Clinic Staff, Jan 5, 2007, Mayo Foundation for Medical Education and Research (http://www.mayoclinic.com/health/performance-enhancing-drugs/SM00045)*
15. *http://www.dallasnews.com/s/dws/spe/2005/steroids/index.html*

Chapter Thirteen

SUPERFOODS, SUPER SUPPLEMENTS

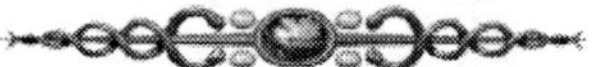

The marketplace is brimming with a wide variety of nutritional products and nutritional supplements. Learning how to best supplement your child's diet is critical today because our food is so depleted of nutrients. In fact, supplementing your child's diet is one of your best investments. You can avert many a doctor's visit, sail through the holidays with no colds or flues, and experience a renewed sense of well being for your whole family.

Superfoods - Simple Solutions

Certain special foods pack an exceptional nutrient punch, more than our daily fare. These "superfoods" are very nutrient-rich, with the ability to fill the nutritional gaps created by our very SAD, Standard American Diet. Superfoods offer:

- Vitamins, minerals, amino acids and fatty acids that improve overall health
- Support for the immune system
- Protection of the body from excess environmental toxins
- The benefit of alkalizing and energizing our cells to balance the body's pH

I recommend that parents incorporate these superfoods into their children's daily food intake. Discuss with your health practitioner which ones are the best for your child:

Colostrum is a powerful infection fighter against bacteria, viruses, fungus and parasites. It is an integral component of mother's milk. Most commercial colostrum is cow-derived, so, it is imperative to use a source from organically-fed cows with no artificial hormones or antibiotic residues. Colostrum is excellent for children with asthma, allergies, yeast infections, eczema or ear infections because it contains active immunoglobulin, lactoferrin and transfer factor for immune support.[1,2]

Lecithin, found in eggs, bee pollen, or soy is often eaten in the form of granules or powder. It is pleasant enough to eat right off the spoon, on top of cereal or oatmeal, or in a smoothie. It is excellent for nourishing the membranes of the brain as it contains the phospholipid, phosphatidylcholine, which supplies the body with two B vitamins, choline and inositol. These are both very important nutrients for the brain cells because they enhance neurotransmitter production. Increasing levels of the neurotransmitter, acetylcholine in the brain, choline and inositol help sharpen the memory process as well as the rate of learning.[3]

Tocotrienols in the form of powdered rice bran is rich with mega-antioxidant qualities, as well as cholesterol-lowering properties. It is excellent for bowel health. New research points to tocotrienols impacting the cardiovascular system. Tocotrienols are a major component of vitamin E and can also be found in palm oil and the annatto seed, harvested in South America.[4,5] It is quite pleasant-tasting, rather nutty, and can be used as a topping for cereals, yogurt, or straight off the spoon.

Aloe is a powerful intestinal, immune and skin healer for the "inside skin" or digestive tract, as well as the external skin. It is available in liquid, powder or capsule form and is helpful for constipation, acid reflux, leaky gut syndrome, eczema and psoriasis. It can also be used topically on rashes, cuts or burns. Add it to water, juice, or a smoothie.

Whey is a great source of protein or amino acids for all ages, from infancy to adulthood. A protein in milk products, cow whey is the most popular, but goat whey contains more minerals. It may also be less allergic. Whey can be easily purchased from your health food store or your health practitioner, and mixed with water, juice, applesauce or yogurt, as well as in a shake or smoothie. It is a favorite of body builders for enhancing muscle growth and has been found to be very therapeutic for infants with colic.[6]

Raw Sprouts represent a big array of nutrients, wrapped in little packages. The two most common types of sprouts are alfalfa and mung bean.

- Alfalfa sprouts, often thought to be a grass, are really a type of lentil and belong to the pea family. Their roots reach between 10 - 30 feet, farther into the soil than any other vegetable! Because they reach deeply for vitamins and minerals, they are extremely nutrient-rich. Alfalfa sprouts are used primarily in salads (often found in salad bars) and on sandwiches.
- Mung bean sprouts, with their high water and mineral content, are an integral part of Asian cooking and can also be used in salads.
- Sprouts with high-antioxidant properties are buckwheat, broccoli, adzuki, clover, garbanzo, lentil, soybean, radish, and my favorite - the juicy and

delectable sunflower sprout. They can be a great addition to sandwiches or can be blended in a food processor and added to smoothies, puddings and other foods for a super nutrient boost!

Raw seeds contain essential fatty acids, amino acids, vitamins and minerals. Popular varieties are sunflower, pumpkin, hemp and flax. They can be eaten in whole, raw form or can be ground and sprinkled in food or a smoothie.

ORAC or Oxygen Radical Absorption Capacity foods have been tested and scored for their ORAC or antioxidant power. Thus, high ORAC foods are particularly potent in their ability to protect the immune system and help slow the aging process of the body and the brain. This is pertinent for children today, as they are bombarded with damaging toxins in our food, air and water. Including high ORAC foods in their diet may protect children from early disease and organ degeneration.

- ORAC foods can also be important for children and adults with asthma and respiratory problems, as they protect the capillaries in the lungs from oxidative damage.[7] Foods high on the ORAC scoreboard include prunes, raisins, blueberries, blackberries, kale, strawberries, spinach, raspberries, Brussels sprouts, plums, alfalfa sprouts and broccoli flowers. According to an ORAC analysis, acai, a small black coconut from the palm tree, which is harvested in the Brazilian rainforest, is an unusually potent ORAC food.

Bee Pollen was first recorded as being used as far back as 2735 B.C. and has always been a powerful source of nutrients. It contains the B complex vitamins, including folic acid, as well as vitamins C, E, A and the carotenoids. Bee pollen also provides a rich variety of minerals, trace nutrients and essential fatty acids. It is especially therapeutic for the reproductive, immune and nervous systems. It helps strengthen blood cell walls and capillaries, and prevents free radical damage to the cells. Good for anemia and high blood pressure, bee pollen is a favorite among athletes looking to improve endurance and strength. It can also be used to help eliminate food cravings, allergies and infections.

Royal Jelly or "bee's milk" is well known for its ability to support the immune system. The queen bee's only food source, this dynamic food is responsible for turning an ordinary worker bee into a long-lived reproductive queen. The queen bee grows 40-60 percent larger than her worker bees and lives for up to 5 full years, whereas her counterpart lives for only 5 months! Royal jelly also contains 22 amino acids and notable quantities of calcium, copper, iron and potassium.

Bee Propolis for human use dates back over 2000 years. Rich in bioflavonoids including quercetin, propolis contains all the known vitamins (except K) and 14 of the 15 minerals (except sulfur). Bee propolis has long been known to have natural antibiotic properties. It has been documented as effective against parasites, fungal infections and viruses, especially herpes and influenza. Studies have also shown that propolis extracts inhibit tumor cell growth and boost the body's T-cell counts.[8]

Chlorophyll is an internal and external healer, used as an antiseptic, heavy metal chelator and blood builder. In liquid or powder form, chlorophyll can be taken in water, juice or in smoothies. *Remember, when you're green inside, you're clean inside!*

Cereal Grasses are a group that includes wheat grass, barley grass and alfalfa. They are harvested in the reproductive cycle before the grain is produced, so they are rich in vitamins and minerals, comparable to dark green vegetables. They are pressed for their juice and packaged as powder, capsules and tablets. Thankfully, they do not contain allergic compounds, such as gluten, that the grains do. Wheatgrass is known for its immune-enhancing qualities. Barley grass is a strong antioxidant food with high amounts of beta carotene, vitamins B and C, and minerals. Alfalfa is considered to be the richest source of land minerals.

The Algae Family consists of about 30,000 different unicellular and multi-cellular species. They proliferate in water: oceans, lakes and, yes, even your pool. We are interested in health benefits of several different forms of food-grade algae. Here are some interesting facts about algae:

- Produces 80 percent of the world's oxygen
- Plays a significant role in climatic change and weather control
- Helps establish the ozone layer
- Is an important component of topsoil
- Sits on the bottom of the food chain, where the most energy is consolidated
- Helps provide safe alternatives for fuel, fertilizer, pesticides
- Is eaten by natives and astronauts alike because of its high nutrient content

Below is a description of several popular algal species used as food or nutritional supplements:

Seaweeds or sea vegetables are the largest and most complex marine or salt water forms of algae. They are photosynthetic, like plants, but simpler because they lack the many of the distinct organs found in land plants. They are really neither plants nor animals, but marine macro-algae, and are classified by color: brown, red, and green.

Seaweeds were an ancient form of food, harvested and eaten long before land-based agriculture. They contain virtually all of the minerals found in the ocean, which are almost the exact same concentration of minerals found in healthy human blood.

They are an excellent source of iodine, magnesium and folate, and a good source of iron, calcium, riboflavin and pantothenic acid. The most common forms of seaweed are dulse, hijiki, kelp, kombu, nori and wakame. Dulse and kelp are rich sources of iodine, beneficial for healthy thyroid function. Nori is probably the seaweed your kids would be most familiar with, as it is used in making sushi rolls.

Dunaliella, a reddish-colored, green microalgal species, is mass cultivated and has the highest level of beta-carotene, but the lowest protein and chlorophyll content of the food-grade algae. It is well documented for its anti-cancer properties.[9]

Chlorella is a small, one-celled fresh-water green algae. It contains more chlorophyll and less protein than other algae and has an indigestible cell wall, which must be "cracked" in order to be absorbed. Widely eaten in Japan, it is used to protect from radiation and highly toxic air pollution. Its popularity is ever increasing, especially in its use for chelation of toxic metals from the body. It can be especially effective in helping to detoxify mercury poisoning from dental amalgams or toxic seafood. It is available in capsule or powder form from your health food store or your health care practitioner.

Spirulina is a species of spiral-shaped blue-green algae, mostly cultivated in man-made lakes or ponds. It is the most domesticated and farmed commercial algae, and probably the most popularly consumed. Spirulina is very rich in antioxidants. Its beta carotene content is ten times that of carrots. Other antioxidants contained in spirulina, zeaxanthin and lutein, are especially good for the eyes.

Spirulina is currently being studied as an excellent food for the rapid recovery from malnutrition and related diseases around the world. It has many therapeutic properties. With its high antioxidant content, it has been found to improve immune function and relieve and prevent hay fever.[10] It has also been shown to reduce the severity of strokes and improve recovery of movement after a stroke.[11] Additionally, spirulina can help to reverse age-related decline in memory and learning.[12]

Aphanizomenon flos aquae or AFA Blue Green Algae is a unique species of algae, harvested in the wild from Klamath Lake, Oregon. It has the capacity to synthesize far greater than many other organisms. Consequently, it contains three times as much chlorophyll as alfalfa, which is why it is referred to as "green blood".

Over three billion years old, AFA algae have adapted to and survived extreme changes in the environment. They are one of the richest plant sources of beta carotene and have a highly assimilable form of B12. They have a high ORAC value. AFA algae also possess a uniquely-balanced fatty acid profile of Omega - 3's and - 6's, as well as many trace minerals, commonly deficient in our food supply: boron, chromium, sulfur, titanium, vanadium and zinc.

This species of algae has an extremely balanced amino acid profile, which provides neuro-peptides that help build our brains' neurotransmitters. This allows the nerve cells to communicate at peak capacity with the rest of the body, positively affecting behavior and emotions. It is most commonly used in capsule or powder form.

The brain-enhancing qualities of AFA are well documented in Dr. Jeffrey Bruno's *Edible Microalgae*: "A Review of the Health Research". Dr. Bruno cites research in Japan, Israel, the Netherlands, and the United States, demonstrating the positive effects of blue green algae on brain function: improved cognition, mood, behavior and academic performance".[13,14]

As shown below, AFA blue green algae have many other documented benefits:

Blue Green Algae (AFA) Helps with Attention and Learning
"Effects of Blue Green Algae Aphanizomenon flos-aquae on 142 children, ages 3-17, struggling with attention, learning or language difficulties, " Jarrett C, The Children and Algae Report, Center For Family Wellness, Harvard, Mass., 1996

"Eating Aphanizomenon flos-aquae triggers highly significant improvement in areas of focus, concentration, family and social interactions, creativity and a decrease in aggressive and "acting out" behaviors."

Blue-Green Algae Improves Nutrition and School Performance
"Study on the Effects of AFA algae on the Nutritional Status and School Performance of First, Second and Third Grade Children Attending the Mosenor Velez School in Nandaime, Nicaragua", Sevilla, I, Aguirre, N, The Nicaragua Report, July 1995

Over 1,561 students were fed blue green algae over a 2-year period. The students' grades increased from 64% to 80.4%. Their attendance increased from 89% to 97%. This school became the highest achieving school in Nicaragua on SAT scores. Also, malnutrition reduced in the students and they became ill less frequently.

Lowered aluminum, with better detoxification and improved cognitive, behavioral ratings by children eating Aphanizomenon flos-aquae.
Bruno J, Gittelman J, Tuchfeld B. Submitted for publication, 2000.

A class of special reading students was fed blue green algae and had significant improvement in behavior, attention, concentration, memory and health symptoms. Also, high levels of toxic metals, uranium, lead and aluminum found in the students' hair were eliminated and the levels normalized as a result of the algae program.

Consumption of Aphanizomenon flos-aquae has Rapid Effects on the Circulation and Function of Immune Cells in Humans.
Jensen, G et al. (2000), Journal of the American Nutraceutical Association 2(3):50-58

AFA (freshwater blue-green algae) increases the immune surveillance without directly stimulating the immune system. These data support signaling from the gut or GI tract to the Central Nervous System to the lymph tissue (part of the immune system).

Effects of AFA Blue-Green Algae on Human Natural Killer Cells
Manoukian, R, et al, 1998 Royal Victoria Hospital, Montreal, Optimal Health Report

"In a double blind, cross-over study ... it was discovered that eating AFA algae triggered the migration of 40% of the circulating Natural Killer (NK) cells from the blood to the tissue within 2 hours."
Some of the NK cells that remained in the bloodstream had 2-3 times as many adhesion molecules as they did before the blue green algae was eaten. The AFA algae strongly triggers movement of NK cells, so vital to destruction of viral and cancer cells.

Algae May Improve Cholesterol Levels
Kushak, RJ, Drapeau, C, Van Cott, EM, et al, Journ of Amer Nutraceut Assoc, vol. 2, No. 3, 2000, pp. 59-65

AFA Algae contain polyunsaturated fatty acids (or PUFA's) and, thus, may have cholesterol-lowering properties, making it a valuable nutritional resource.

Bioregulatory and Therapeutic Effects of Blue Green Algae
Kumar, K, Lakshmanan, A, Kannaiyan, S, Indian JNL of Microbiology, 2003, vol. 43, no1, pp. 9-16

A water based extract of Aphanizomenon flos-aquae containing high concentrations of phycocyanin, a virucidal protein, inhibited the in vitro growth of 1 out of 4 tumor cell lines, indicating that some tumor cell types may be sensitive to killing by phycocyanin.

AFA blue-green algae products are available from your health practitioner, your health food store or from www.simplexityhealth.com.

Brain Nutrients & Supplements

The brain requires fuel for proper functioning: water, oxygen, glucose and other nutrients from our food. Many nutritional supplements, vitamins, minerals, herbs, fatty acids and amino acids can cover these bases. Here is what they assist in:

- Growth and repair of brain and nerve cells
- Protection of brain and nerve cells
- Fluidity and flexibility of the membranes of each cell
- Production of neurotransmitters or brain chemicals
- Balance or homeostasis of the body

The following pages reveal just some of the key nutrients that can accomplish these tasks.

Herbs

(Note: Always check with your doctor before combining herbs with prescription medications or over-the-counter drugs.)

Bacopa monniera improves memory function and has been shown to increase neurotransmitters, especially serotonin. It has been used to ease anxiety, depression, dementia, hyperactivity, focus and concentration problems.

Centella asiatica is considered a nerve and brain tonic, known to increase memory.

Chamomile is a well-known component of tea for sleep time. It is also used to relieve headaches, anxiety and pain.

Ginkgo Biloba is an herb that enhances blood circulation and increases oxygen supply to the brain and body. It increases the rate of nerve transmissions, improves production of neurotransmitters and enhances neurotransmitter receptors in the brain's memory center, the hippocampus. Thus, it enhances memory.

A series of studies testing cerebral insufficiency with symptoms of short-term memory loss and lack of alertness have shown incredible improvements of 44% to 92%, with use of ginkgo.[15] Also mono amino oxidase (MAO) is a compound that breaks down neurotransmitters and contributes to depression. Some anti-depressant drugs are called MAO inhibitors. Ginkgo is a natural MAO inhibitor.

Another study, based on increasing blood flow to certain regions of the brain, used a combination of ginkgo and ginseng for a positive affect on children: between one third and three quarters of the children experienced reduced anxiety, shyness, social problems, hyperactivity, and/or impulsiveness.[16]

American Ginseng or Panax quinquefolius is an adaptogenic herb that helps the body handle stress and reverse fatigue. It has also been found to improve focus and concentration. There are many types of ginseng but the other popular one is called:

Gotu Kola or Hydrocotyle Asiatica fortifies the immune system and strengthens the adrenal glands. In Ayurvedic medicine, it is used to treat insomnia, nervousness, and senility, and promote clarity, better memory and concentration.[17]

Hops is an herb that has long been used to help with insomnia and anxiety.

Passion Flower has a sedative effect and is often found in formulations used to relieve anxiety, hyperactivity and insomnia.

Pycnogenol is a trade name for proanthocyanidins, which are bioflavonoids. It is derived from grape seed or pine bark extract and has been used with great success to decrease symptoms of ADD and ADHD by improving circulation to the brain.[18] It is available in capsule form.

Siberian ginseng (Eleutherococcus senticosus) is really not of the ginseng family, but bears the same name. It is from Russia, is less expensive and believed to have identical benefits.

Skullcap can help alleviate anxiety and restlessness. It helps promote muscle relaxation and sleep.

Schizandra is an adaptogenic herb used quite a bit in Chinese medicine as a stress reliever and adrenal gland fortifier. Thus, it helps to improve brain efficiency, increase work capacity and build strength. It is said to reduce the negative effects of caffeine.

St. John's Wort is a well-studied herbal anti-depressant and pain reliever.[19] Speak with your doctor or pediatrician before combining it with prescription medications.

Valerian is often used in the treatment of nervous conditions including hysteria, hypochondria, nervous unrest and emotional troubles. It is most widely known as a calming agent, beneficial for sleep disorders. It is available in capsule or tincture form.

Wild Oats or Avena Sativa is one of the best herbs for nourishing the nervous system and is recommended to relieve exhaustion, depression and the effects of stress.

Vitamins

B Complex Vitamins are vital for maintaining the nerve cells and buffering stress.

B1 or Thiamine is a B vitamin that has long been studied for its ability to increase capacity for learning. It has also been used in psychiatric patients to reduce symptoms of manic depression.

Folic Acid or Folate or B2 is vitally important for development, transmission and repair of nerve and brain cells. It helps with circulation, memory and cognitive function.

B3 or Niacin is a B vitamin that stimulates circulation in the brain and helps enhance memory.

NADH, derived from niacin, helps alleviate depression. It is involved in the synthesis of ATP (adenosine triphosphate), the body's primary source of intracellular energy. It also supports cell regulation, DNA repair, antioxidant activity and the production of brain chemicals, adrenaline, dopamine, serotonin and norepinephrine.

Choline is a B vitamin that helps build acetylcholine, a neurotransmitter. It is vital for proper transmission of the nerve impulses from the brain through the entire nervous system. Choline is available in supplement form and is found in lecithin, egg yolks, liver, meat, fish, legumes, cauliflower, cabbage, soybeans and whole grain cereals.

Inositol is choline's partner. The two are often found together in foods and supplements. An important component of lecithin, inositol is essential for fat metabolism. Known for its calming effect on the nervous system, it is utilized in nutritional supplements that enhance sleep. Additionally, it helps reduce cholesterol.

DMAE is a compound that is closely related to choline and helps to improve memory by aiding in the production of acetylcholine. It is known to elevate moods and create emotional balance. It has helped many children "with" ADD, especially those without hyperactivity. DMAE is found in anchovies, sardines and other fish.

B5 or Pantothenic Acid is often used in adrenal formulas, because it helps produce the adrenal hormones, adrenaline and cortisol. Consequently, it is known to enhance energy and balance stress. A deficiency may lead to fatigue, headaches, tingling in the extremities or constipation.

B6 or Pyridoxine is involved in more activities in the body than almost any other nutrient. For brain function, it is most known for its calming effect, memory enhancement and cognitive improvement. It is also used in formulas for anti-anxiety and relief of insomnia. It is found in Brewer's yeast, eggs, chicken, fish, meat, peas, cabbage, sunflower seeds and walnuts.

B12 or Methylcobalamin or Cyanocobalamin plays very important roles in brain and nerve cell function. It prevents nerve damage, assists in memory and learning and protects the nerve endings by promoting normal development of the fatty sheaths. It helps prevent memory loss and depression and supports energy production.

Co Enzyme Q10 is related to the B vitamin family and is found in every cell in the body. For this reason, it is called "ubiquinone" or "found everywhere". Its highest concentrations are in the heart, liver and muscles. It is required for the production of energy in every cell. Co Q 10 energizes the brain and strengthens the immune system, making it vital for people with allergies and cancer, especially breast cancer. Co Q10 studies are especially focused in the areas of cardiovascular and heart strengthening, lung and respiratory enhancement, prevention of gum disease and improved athletic performance.[20,21]

Better energy, muscle strength and endurance are reported by many people who take Co Q 10. It is often helpful for children with asthma, allergies, ADD and ADHD. Present in many of whole grains, Co Q10 has been milled away in most grain-based processed foods, flour products and baked goods. It is now deficient in our food supply, but thankfully available in liquid or capsule form.

Vitamin C is the most popular and highly studied vitamin for its immune and strong anti-viral properties. It is an antioxidant, protecting from free radical damage of brain cells and the spinal cord.

Minerals

Calcium, the most abundant mineral in the body, builds and maintains bones and teeth. It regulates heart rhythm and eases insomnia. Calcium maintains proper nerve, muscle and kidney function. A deficiency can result in muscle spasms, cramps, soft or brittle bones, slow growth, tooth decay, fidgetiness and hyper behavior.

Magnesium is a mineral, which is potentially involved in over 300 enzymatic reactions in the body. It plays a crucial role in regulating the neuromuscular activity of the heart, maintaining normal heart rhythm and converting blood sugar into energy. It is calming for the nervous system. Deficiency of magnesium can result in calcium depletion, heart spasms, nervousness, confusion, muscle cramps and kidney stones.

Lithium is a mineral found naturally in seaweed, potatoes, lemon and certain mineral waters. It can be concentrated in capsule form as lithium orotate or can be used as a homeopathic for therapeutic purposes. (Do not confuse this with the prescription drug, Lithium.) Natural lithium has been found to be an effective mood stabilizer. It acts to decrease norepinphrine, the brain chemical that can cause anxiety. It can be helpful for those with mood swings, manic depression and bi-polar disorder.[22]

Zinc (No Zinc, No Think!) Zinc is a mineral that is utilized in many of the body's processes: digestion, immune enhancement, adrenal function, pancreatic function, brain function and multitude of other metabolic processes. A zinc deficiency may lead to problems with appetite, growth, skin, immune health and cognitive processes. Many children, especially those "with ADD and ADHD" are deficient in zinc.

Here are some of zinc's properties:

- Stimulates mental activity
- Regulates appetite (in anorexia and bulimia) and taste disorders
- Improves muscle strength and endurance
- Strengthens white blood cells; increases response to injury & infection
- Essential for rapid cell division, as in the developing fetus. Research has shown that growing children and pregnant women require more zinc per pound than the rest of the population.
- Helps to balance growth disorders
- Improves adrenal function to balance energy and stress
- Increases wound healing
- Helps to correct skin disorders
- Helps in the manufacture of body's hormones and brain chemicals

Checking for zinc deficiency is easy when using a special zinc taste test. If you drink a special zinc liquid and it tastes like water, you are deficient. If it tastes horrible, you're not deficient. Many kids, especially those with ADHD have zinc deficiencies. (Call 800-608-5602 for this zinc taste test.)

Zinc is most available to the body from plant-based foods, seafood, meat, rice, beans, unprocessed cereals, unprocessed cheeses, seeds and nuts.

Amino Acids

Amino acids provide building materials for neurotransmitters and can also work as brain chemicals themselves. Freshwater blue green algae and whey protein are excellent sources of amino acids. Amino acids are also available individually or in combinations, as capsules from your health food store or your health practitioner.

5-HPT or 5-Hydroxytryptophan is a precursor to serotonin, which means that serotonin is manufactured from 5-HTP in the brain and in the intestinal tract. This nutrient can be impactful for relieving anxiety, depression, poor appetite, hyperactivity and insomnia. It is available in powder or capsule form from your health practitioner.[23]

Acetyl-L-Carnitine supports awareness and thought processes (cognition) by increasing neural metabolism, supporting the activity of neurotransmitters, serotonin and dopamine and enhancing cerebral blood flow.[24] It aids in the conversion of fat for cellular energy and is available in capsule form.

GABA (Gamma-amino-butyric-acid) is a neurotransmitter than aids in the production of serotonin. GABA and serotonin can be helpful in enhancing focus and concentration, as well as calming anxiety and hyperactivity. Insomnia may also be relieved with GABA. It is available in capsule form and can be opened up and added to juice or food.

Glutamic Acid is fuel for the brain and important for the production of GABA.

L-Glutamine is an amino acid which readily enters the brain and is used for energy and the manufacture of brain chemicals. It is also a precursor to glutathione, which is important to help the body detoxify. It is found in capsule or powder form in various supplements for brain power, as well as healing the GI tract.

L-Glycine is an amino acid that helps to buffer electrical and chemical transmissions in the brain. It is also a building block for glutathione.

Phenylalanine is an essential amino acid that aids in the production of the neurotransmitter norepinephrine, promoting mental alertness, vitality, improved learning and memory. It is also important because it converts to tyrosine and supports thyroid function.

SAMe or S-Adenosyl-Methionine (SAMe) is involved in regulating the brain's neurotransmitters, serotonin and epinephrine. Normally the brain manufactures all the SAMe it needs from the amino acid methionine, unless a person has a low protein diet or malabsorption problems. SAMe, in supplement form, has been studied for its effects in lifting depression and assisting in the production of endorphins which block pain.[25,26]

Taurine is an amino acid and an antioxidant for the brain. A neurotransmitter or brain chemical in its own right, taurine helps prevent brain over-activity, assists in the regulation of heartbeat and is an important component of bile which helps digest fats. Taurine is found in meat and fish and is available in nutritional supplement form.

Tyrosine is an amino acid that helps build the brain chemicals, norepinephrine and dopamine, which help lift depression and improve cognitive function. Tyrosine is required to produce the thyroid hormones that balance metabolism and burn calories.

Lipids and Fats

DHA (docosahexaenoic acid) is important from both structural and functional points-of-view for brain health. Remember that the brain is made of 60 percent fats, and DHA is 25 percent of that.[27,28] Cod liver oil and other fish oils are noted for containing DHA, the major fatty acid required for eye, brain, nerve and heart tissue health. It is also contained in some micro-algae, wild salmon, herring and tuna.

Research points to DHA deficiencies in children and adults with ADD and ADHD.[29] Although DHA can be manufactured from other fats, like Omega-3 oils, some people's bodies have difficulty in this conversion process. Why not get the DHA straight from the food source? Use cod liver oil or blue-green algae for a direct source.

EPA (eicosapentaenoic acid) is often coupled with DHA, as the 2 Omega-3 fatty acids occur together in the fish oils from cod, salmon, krill and sardines. EPA/DHA supplements are popular for children with ADD, ADHD and autism, as they have been proven in studies to help develop and enhance brain and cognitive function. (See studies in C*hapter 2*.)

Phospholipids such as phosphatidylcholine and phosphatidylserine are fats that are incorporated into the membranes of the neurons or nerve cells. These are constantly being replaced due to normal wear and tear --- thinking and life's activities. They are vitally important for children who exhibit signs of hyperactivity, depression, lack of focus, lack of concentration, allergies, and asthma or skin problems.

As stated earlier, phosphatidylcholine supplies the body with two B vitamins, choline and inositol, which enhance the production of the neurotransmitters or brain chemicals. In particular, it helps boost acetylcholine in the brain, which sharpens the memory process and the rate of learning.

In his book, *Phosphatidylserine*, Dr. Parris Kidd notes that at least 64 human studies have been published on "PS". Consistent positive findings establish that "PS" can help with depression, insomnia, stress relief and revitalizing an "aging" brain.[30]

"PS" helps boost alpha brain waves, inducing calmness. It assists in fact and number recall and increases concentration while reading. Phospholipids are found in soy, soy lecithin, eggs and bee pollen. They can be taken in powder, liquid or capsule form.

Ideas for Feeding Supplements to Children

For Infants:

If mom is breastfeeding, she can ingest the nutrients in order to get them to the child via the breast milk. If the child is on a formula part of the time or all the time, the capsules can be opened up or tablets can be ground up and added to the formula.

For Toddlers:

If the child is eating food, the liquid, powder or capsule supplements can be added to applesauce, oatmeal, fruit juices diluted with water, vegetables or baby food. Parents are pretty inventive and have used the following ideas:

- A dropper or a baby syringe filled with the appropriate nutrients or supplements in a liquid medium can be inserted in the child's mouth. For some toddlers, this may be a simpler approach.
- A small shot glass can be used with the ingredients of an opened-up capsule, topped off with water or a little juice.
- If you use a whole capsule, it can be opened up and emptied into the liquid or food. If only a ¼ or ½ capsule is used, it can opened up, partially emptied and closed again for the next dose.
- Taking liquid through a straw helps some kids drink more and not taste as fully. This can be helpful when the supplement alters the taste of the liquid.
- Cold fluids can cover up not-so-good tastes.

All Children:

A general rule of thumb for children's dosages is ¼ to ½ the adult recommended amount. Smaller children may need to use ¼ the adult recommended amount. Specific dosages for super food supplements are not always necessary, but most people like to have a place to start. For digestive enzymes, bifidus, acidophilus and blue green algae, infants and small children may need to begin with ¼ -½ capsule opened up onto the tongue or into the food.

If the child is old enough to swallow capsules, he or she is probably old enough to start with a complete capsule. Amounts may be altered as the child adapts to the taste and routine, and results are observed.

It is optimal for your child to understand the importance of taking supplements and eating super foods to help their body and brain develop with the highest quality nutrients. Once it's explained, kids understand that because many of our foods are depleted of vitamins and minerals, we need to take a concentrated form of these nutrients, such as the blue green algae or other super foods. This can be explained in much the same way that a parent would explain the importance of a multi-vitamin.

Finally, I'll borrow the advice of one of my five-year old patients. He says that if you talk to the vitamin or nutritional supplement before you take it or as you're swallowing it, you won't have any problems!

Benefits that children relate to are:

- Increased athletic abilities - run faster, better skills and focus
- More strength and endurance
- All pro athletes use nutritional supplements and smoothie or protein drinks
- Fewer colds and flues. "It's a drag to be sick."
- Fewer allergies - less stuffiness and drowsiness, breathe better
- Better growth and strength
- Better focus and easier studying
- Good moods, laugh more
- Less pain and inflammation
- Better skin
- Fewer nightmares, more restful sleep

Helping Children Swallow Supplements

Below are ideas for making supplements palatable if your child resists or can't swallow "pills". Tablets can be crushed, capsules can be opened up and powders can be sprinkled into any of the following items:

- Applesauce
- Gravy
- Hot cereal
- Nut butter and jelly sandwich
- Oatmeal
- Organic almond butter
- Organic peanut butter
- Pear sauce
- Roll in burrito or tortilla
- Roll in egg roll
- Smoothie
- Tahini

Juices, Beverages, Milks, Smooth Foods:

- Almond or Hemp milk
- Berry juices provide good camouflage.
- Carrot, beet, celery, parsley juice or any veg combo
- Frosting (chocolate covers well)
- Fruit smoothie
- Fruit sorbet
- Grape juice covers tastes and colors well.
- Ice cream or ice milk
- Mix with favorite fruit juice and freeze as popsicles
- Natural sodas, colas, root beer
- Orange juice covers tastes well.
- Pudding - Rice milk-based Imagine Puddings or dairy puddings
- Rice milk - Rice Dream
- Soy milk - your favorite brand
- Tomato juice

If using a **blue green algae** capsule, a **greens powder** or a **natural color supplement,** it can be successfully covered up in:

- Black bean burrito
- Broccoli – after steaming
- Carob sauce (use natural sweetener and carob powder)
- Chocolate or carob cow's milk
- Chocolate/carob frosting
- Chocolate/carob ice cream
- Chocolate/carob pudding
- Chocolate/carob rice milk
- Chocolate/carob soy milk
- Green beans with sauce
- Guacamole
- Jellies or jams, red or purple
- Peas with a sauce
- Pesto sauce on rice or pasta
- Smoothie/berries for flavor & color
- Soup - after heating
- Spinach – after sautéing

Results That Kids Report

- Balanced moods
- Better ability to communicate
- Better athletic performance
- Better behavior, better grades
- Better bowel movements: no constipation; no diarrhea
- Better breathing, fewer respiratory problems
- Better hearing
- Better memory
- Better mental clarity, attention and focus
- Better muscle tone & coordination
- Better sleep
- Clear skin: improvement with acne, eczema, psoriasis
- Feeling of more acceptance; feeling less weird, more friends
- Fewer colds and flues
- Fewer cravings and addictions
- Happier
- Improved hand-eye coordination
- Improved handwriting
- Less bed-wetting
- Less fidgety
- Less frequent crying or temper tantrums
- Less hyper, more balanced energy
- Less sibling rivalry
- No ear infections
- No gastric disturbances or acid reflux; no indigestion
- No joint pain
- No yeast overgrowth: better skin, less asthma, no fungal,
- Reduced or no allergies
- Reduced thrush or ear infections
- Vitality upon awakening

If you don't get your desired results, here's what to try:

1. Increase water consumption.
2. Speak to a health care professional who has studied nutritional supplements. Ask for his or her advice about amount or potencies of nutritional supplements for your children.

3. Give supplements at different time of day. Try with meals; try without meals.
4. Take advantage of weekends, vacations and summers to experiment when your child is home more.
5. Increase exercise or physical activity to get the blood and lymph systems circulating better.
6. If the child is on medication, talk to your doctor about altering the dosages. It may be important for progress to be made. When the body is nourished and supported naturally, the need for medication often decreases over time.
7. Check for toxic metals through hair analysis. These and other fat-soluble toxins may take longer for the body to eliminate or detoxify, thereby halting noticeable progress.
8. Check for food allergies. Try the rotation diet mentioned in *Chapter 11.*
9. Look for other health-limiting factors:
    a. nail biting, nose picking – may indicate parasitic involvement
    b. continued ingestion of sugar and sweets
    c. continued ingestion of hidden chemicals in foods (Feingold Diet)
10. Look for change of health condition: Sometimes old problems return. For example, if you're looking for more balanced, consistent energy, your body may exhibit other changes first. You may get very tried for a few days or your old eczema problem may re-appear. You wonder, "Why is this happening? I thought I was supposed to be feeling better, not worse." Well, sometimes the body retraces symptoms or conditions as it is healing or coming into balance and you may experience emergence of an old problem. Like a visitor, it is just "passing through" and will generally clear fairly quickly.

It is not uncommon for various health conditions to be rooted in the same cause. They just take on a different picture. If the asthma began after eczema appeared originally, then it may retrace its steps and "go out the way it came in". "Retracing" has been observed by many cultures in the world for centuries -- in India, China and Japan. It is central to the philosophy of naturopathic medicine practiced in Europe, Canada and the U.S. The body has a logic and priority list of its own. We don't always heal in a way that is predictable.

Sometimes other problems clear up first. For instance, if depression resulted from hypoglycemia or a blood sugar imbalance, the blood sugar problem may clear up before the depression disappears. In other words, progress is being made; it's just not obvious to you. A behavior or emotional problem may clear up after you see physical improvements.

Be patient. Turning around behavior and health conditions naturally, takes time.

Pay-off for Parents

It is common for parents to be worried or anxious about their children's health. Following our optimal programs can certainly have a lasting impact on your child, but also, your entire family.

The following are potential benefits:

- Calm family meals
- Cooperation
- Even-tempers and less stress
- Family outings would be fun again
- Fewer doctor's visits
- Fewer family feuds
- Guilt-free time for yourself
- Happy kids, happy parents
- Less physical and emotional pain
- No more embarrassment
- Peace at home
- Peace in the classroom
- Sense of well-being
- Uplifted spirits

Your child will be able to sleep thru the night and you will too. You will then be well rested and encouraged to deal with family challenges as they come, with much less stress. Parents want their children to succeed and it is far easier when they are healthy and feel well.

---

1. *Elrod, KC, et al. "Lactoferrin, a potent striptease inhibitor, abolished late-phase airway responses in allergic sheep," American Journal of Respiratory Critical Care Medicine 156:375-381 (1997).*
2. *Acosta-Altamirano, G, et al. "Anti-amoebic properties of human colostrum," Advances in Experimental Medicine and Biology 216B:1347-1352 (1987). In addition to its effectiveness against bacterial, viral and fungal infections, colostrum also provides protection against amoebic pathogens.*

3. *"Lecithin consumption increases acetylcholine concentrations in rat brain and adrenal gland", Science 13 October 1978: Vol. 202. no. 4364, pp. 223 – 225, DOI: 10.1126/science.694529*
4. *Supplementary tocotrienols exert antioxidant effects in humans and help stabilize arterial capacity for normal blood flow, Lipids, 1995; 30: 1179-83.*
5. *Qureshi AA and Qureshi N, Tocotrienols: Novel hypocholesterolemic agents with antioxidant properties. In L. Packer and J. Fuchs (ed.), Vitamin E in Health and Disease. Marcel Dekker, 1993, New York.*
6. *Lucassen PL, et al. Infantile colic: crying time reduction with a whey hydrolysate: a double-blind, randomized, placebo-controlled trial. Pediatrics, December 6, 2000; 106: 1349-54.*
7. *"Can Foods Forestall Aging?", McBride, J, Agricultural Research Magazine, February 1999, United States Department of Agriculture.*
8. *Guarini L, Su ZZ, Zucker S, Lin J, Grunberger D, and Fisher PB, "Growth inhibition and modulation of antigenic phenotype in human melanoma and glioblastoma multiform cells by caffecic acid phenethyl ester (CAPE)", Cellular Molecular Biology, 38 (5) 1992*
9. *Bruno, J, PhD, Edible Microalgae: A Review of the Health Research, Center for Nutritional Psychology Press, 2001, p. 177.*
10. *.Chen, LL, et al. "Experimental study of spirulina platensis in treating allergic rhinitis in rats." Journal of Central South University (Medical Sciences). Feb. 2005. 30(1):96-8.*
11. *Wang, Y., et al. "Dietary supplementation with blueberries, spinach, or spirulina reduces ischemic brain damage." Experimental Neurology. May, 2005; 193(1):75-84.*
12. *Gemma, C., et al. "Diets enriched in foods with high antioxidant activity reverse age-induced decreases in cerebellar beta-adrenergic function and increases in pro-inflammatory cytokines." Experimental Neurology. July 15, 2002; 22(14):6114-20.*
13. *Edible Microalgae: A Review of the Health Research, Bruno, J, PhD, Center for Nutritional Psychology Press, 2001*
14. *Bruno, J, PhD, Edible Microalgae: A Review of the Health Research, Center for Nutritional Psychology Press, 2001*
15. *Becker M. Ginkgo biloba. Proc UCLA Health 2000 Spring; 4(1):40-1.*
16. *Lyon MR, Cline JC, Totosy de Zepetnek J, Shan JJ, Pang P, Benishin C. "Effect of the herbal extract combination Panax quinquefolium & Ginkgo biloba on attention-deficit hyperactivity disorder: a pilot study." J Psychiatry Neurosci. 2001 May; 26(3):221-8.*
17. *Veerendra Kumar MH, Gupta YK. Effect of Centella asiatica on cognition and oxidative stress in an intracerebroventricular streptozotocin model of Alzheimer's disease in rats. Clin Exp Pharmacol Physiol. 2003 May-Jun; 30(5-6):336-42.*
18. *Rohdewald P. "A review of the French maritime pine bark extract (Pycnogenol), a herbal medication with a diverse clinical pharmacology", Int J Clin Pharmacol Ther. 2002 Apr; 40(4):158-68.*

19. *Clement, K, Covertson, CR, Johnson MJ, Dearing K. "St. John's Wort and the treatment of mild to moderate depression: A systematic review." Holistic Nurse Pract. 2006 Jul-Aug: 20(4): 197-203.*
20. *Berman, M., Erman, A., Ben Gal, T., Dvir, D., Georghiou, G. P., Stamler, A., Vered, Y., Vidne, B. A., and Aravot, D. Coenzyme Q10 in patients with end-stage heart failure awaiting cardiac transplantation: a randomized, placebo-controlled study. Clin.Cardiol. 2004; 27(5):295-299.*
21. *Bresolin, N., Doriguzzi, C., Ponzetto, C., Angelini, C., Moroni, I., Castelli, E., Cossutta, E., Binda, A., Gallanti, A., Gabellini, S., & Ubidecarenone in the treatment of mitochondrial myopathies: a multi- center double-blind trial. Journal of Neurol.Sci 1990; 100(1-2):70-78.*
22. *Dean W, English J, ""Lithium Orotate: The Unique, Safe Mineral with Multiple Uses," Vitamin Research News, July, 1999.*
23. *Birdsail, TC, "5-Hydroxytryptophan: a clinically-effective serotonin precursor", Alternative Medicine Review, 1998 Aug:3(4):27*
24. *Tolu P, Masi F, Leggio B, Schleggl S, Tagliamonte A, de Montia MG. Effects of long-term acetyl-L-carnitine in rats: I. Increased dopamine output in mesocorticolimbic areas and protection toward acute stress exposure. Neuropsychopharmacology. 2002 Sep; 27(3):410-20.*
25. *Bressa GM, "S-adenosyl-l-methionine (SAMe) as antidepressant: meta-analysis of clinical studies", Acta Neurol Scand Suppl 1994;154:7-14*
26. *Jacobsen S., Dannekiold-Samsoe B, Andersen RB. "Oral S-adenosylmethionine in primary fibromyalgia. Double-blind clinical evaluation." Scandinavian Journal of Rheumatology. 1991; 20(4):294-302.*
27. *"Brain Boost: The Tuna Sandwich", Psychology Today, April 29, 2005, Sussex Publishers, LLC.*
28. *"Brain Boost: The Tuna Sandwich", Psychology Today, April 29, 2005, Sussex Publishers, LLC*
29. *"Can Attention Deficit-Hyperactivity Disorder Result from Nutritional Deficiency?" Fred Ottoboni, F, MPH, PhD, Ottoboni, A, PhD, Journal of American Physicians and Surgeons, Summer 2003, pp. 58-60.*
30. *Kidd, P., 1995. Phosphatidylserine (PS), A Remarkable Brain Cell Nutrient. Lucas Meyer, Inc, Decator, Il.*

~ ~ ~

PART FOUR – LET THE FUN BEGIN: Putting It All Together

Chapter Fourteen

A 30-DAY GAME PLAN: Re-Designing Life

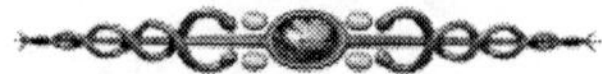

Here is an outline of a 30-day game plan. Use the info in this book to discover alternative ways to implement ideas for healthy eating. This plan can all be adapted to suit your child, family, kitchen, and lifestyle.

Action Steps for Your 30-Day Game Plan

1. Fill out the questionnaire on the next page.
2. Fill out the guideline sheet.
3. Eliminate the offenders, the toxins:
   a. Identify the toxins: preservatives, colorings, pesticides.
   b. Replace them with non-toxic, additive-free, good-tasting foods.
   c. Fill out food diary. Track the food your child is eating, for one week.
   d. Identify allergic foods and eliminate.
4. Buy and consume nutrient-rich food:
   a. Carbohydrates, proteins and fats - organic & unprocessed.
   b. Superfoods such as flax seed oil and wild, freshwater blue green algae are no longer an option; they are a necessity.
5. Ensure optimal digestion and assimilation:
   a. Eat enzymatically active food: organic fruits and vegetables.
   b. Avoid "sludge" foods: fried and fast foods.
   c. Incorporate digestive enzymes and acidophilus in supplement form.
6. Ask important questions. What if your child or teenager could now enjoy:

Better eye contact & awareness
Relief of diarrhea & constipation
Reduced food cravings
Relief of allergies, asthma, eczema
Fewer ear and sinus infections

Better attitude and behavior
Fewer colds and flu
Less absenteeism from school
Balanced energy and vitality

Wouldn't it be worth trying?

This is a program that will help you and your family get back on track. And don't worry, even if you don't follow it exactly, you can still get great benefit. Start your program by filling in the following information.

YOUR HEALTH QUESTIONNAIRE AND GUIDELINE

Printable version on website. www.ourchildrenshealth.com/guidelines

Jot down your answers here or on a separate page. This will help you design a nutrition program that is just right for your children and your family.

Name of child or teen:

Part A: Goals: What improvements would you like to see? Ex: Better behavior, better grades, no colds or flu, better breathing, clear skin, balanced emotions.

1.
2.
3.

Part B: List symptoms: physical, mental, emotional, and behavioral:

Part C: Health History: Has the child or teen had a history of: (check)

- ☐Ear infections?
- ☐Respiratory infections?
- ☐Skin conditions?
- ☐Bed wetting?
- ☐Dry skin?
- ☐Any antibiotics in the past?
- ☐How many rounds?
- ☐Vaccinations?
- ☐Bowel problems?
- ☐Unusual cravings?

List present medications, including over-the-counter:

☐Any surgeries, car accidents, physical traumas?
☐Any dental work or fillings?
Birth/Delivery: ☐Normal ☐C-Section ☐Other ____________

Part D: Elimination and Digestion

☐Bowels move daily?
☐How many?
☐Normal

☐Painful
☐Hard
☐Loose

☐Gas
☐Bloating
☐Cramping

☐Stomach aches
☐Acid reflux

Part E: Behavior and Emotions

Sleep:

☐Hrs per day
☐Restful
☐Restless
☐Difficulty falling asleep

☐Awakes tired
☐Sleepwalks or has nightmares
☐Difficulty staying asleep

Energy Level:

☐Normal
☐Under active
☐Hyper

☐Fidgety
☐Often tired

Learning Challenges?
Diagnosis?
Problems at School?

Behavior at School:

☐Normal
☐Hyperactive
☐Withdrawn
☐Defiant

☐Aggressive
☐Violent
☐Daydreamer
☐Temper tantrums

Emotional State:

☐Happy
☐Depressed

☐Mood swings

Part F: Food Habits, Diet and Nutrition

Do you suspect any food allergies or sensitivities? If so what?
Any environmental allergies or sensitivities? If so what?

☐Genetic predisposition (family members with allergies)?

Intense cravings?

☐Cheese or milk
☐Chips or salty foods
☐Sugar
☐Chocolate
☐Spicy foods
☐Carbohydrates (cereals, breads, pastas)

Food:

☐Fast food
☐Packaged mixes
☐Frozen dinners
☐Canned foods?

Does the child/teen eat natural or health foods? ☐Yes ☐No

Does the child have any dislikes?

☐oz. -- How much water does he/she drink?
☐oz -- How much should he/she drink? (hint: ½ oz. per lb. of body weight)

What other beverages does the child drink?

☐Regular soda
☐Diet soda
☐Gatorade
☐Fruit drinks
☐Real fruit juice
☐Coffee, tea (caffeine)
☐Herbal tea
☐Sports drinks
☐Other caffeinated drinks
☐Milk or milk substitute

Part G: Nutritional Supplements

Does your child/teen take vitamins or other nutritional supplements? List:	

Is the child able to swallow capsules or tablets? ☐Yes ☐No

Guideline Sheet

Use this sheet to list your suggestions, as each part correlates with questionnaire. Check with your health practitioner to validate your assessment.

Part A: Goals
1.
2.
3.

Part B: Symptoms
1.
2.
3.

Part C: Health History
1.
2.
3.

Part D: Elimination and Digestion
1.
2.
3.

Part E: Behavior and Emotions
1.
2.
3.

Part F: Food Habits: Diet and Nutrition
1.
2.
3.

Part G: Nutritional Supplements
1.
2.
3.

Your 30-Day Game Plan
For Improving Behavior, Health, and School Performance

Week 1 Activity 1	Use the completed Health Questionnaire and Guideline Sheet in this chapter. This will help you identify a starting point for beginning your health program project.
Activity 2	The next step for most families is to go through your kitchen cabinets and refrigerator and weed out all the products that contain chemical toxins, food colorings, additives, preservatives, and artificial sweeteners. This process usually takes about two weeks. Sometimes you discover things in stages. Throw or give them away.
Activity 3	Locate your local health food stores, large or small, and food co-ops and farmers' markets where you can buy chemical-free foods and local produce.
Activity 4	Begin to replace these processed foods with purer foods. See Substitution Lists for ideas. Take this book to the store with you, to identify foods and brand names. This is a process, so be patient. You will get the hang of it and the family will find foods that they like.
Activity 5	Good starting point is with breakfast cereals and snack foods. These are major culprits of chemical exposure to children through the colorings, preservatives, additives, and sugar.
Activity 6	Get kids involved in label-reading and even in food preparation. If the child is very young, then involvement might be just stirring or emptying something into a bowl. Give responsibilities accordingly, to instill pride and knowledge about foods and their preparation.
Supplements	Start your child and your family with 1 digestive enzyme capsule with each meal. If the kids can't take an enzyme to school for lunchtime, then make sure to give them an enzyme at breakfast & dinner. If the child is very small you can begin with ½ enzyme capsule per meal.
Notes	All the supplements recommended in this program are useful for infants and very small children as well. They may need to begin their supplement program with ¼ or ½ capsule. Simply open the capsule and add the desired amount into food or a beverage. Suggestions are listed in *Chapter 13: Ideas for Feeding Supplements to Children.*

Week Two:

Activity 1	Read again the *Family Meals Chapter 10* and extract ideas for packed lunches and family dinners that you'd like to try.
Activity 2	Continue weeding out your cabinets and refrigerators. Continue to rotate in purer foods, the ones without the chemicals.
Activity 3	Begin to identify the purest of meats, poultry and seafood. Use these only, once your storage of others runs out.
Activity 4	Continue experimenting with the foods from the Substitution Lists. Begin to utilize breads, cereals, cookies, etc. from grains other than wheat. The quality of carbohydrates will be improved by doing this --less refined and more complex carbohydrates, rendering more balanced, consistent physical and mental energy.
Activity 5	What beverages are your children drinking? Water should be the primary one. (See water chart in *Digestion Chapter 3*.) Reduce milk, juice, and soda intake. Remember, these qualify as foods; only water and herb teas are not foods. Over-ingestion of milk, soda, and juice is a primary cause of hyperactivity, obesity and loss of appetite.
Activity 6	Remember that exercise helps develop better brain function.
Activity 7	Observe whether your child has any food allergies or sensitivities. Remember, they may manifest in various ways: excess mucus congestion, digestive discomfort, gas or bloating, abnormal bowel consistency, acne, eczema, psoriasis, ear infections, mood swings, depression, hyperactivity, irritability, and fatigue. It's possible that one or more food substances may be causing these problems.
Supplements	Continue one enzyme per meal. (1/2 enzyme for smaller kids.) Try a superfood-supplement for enhanced brain or immune function, such as blue green algae. (See *Chapter 13*.)
Notes	Sometimes the body goes through a period of adjustment when you make lots of changes -- putting in the good, pushes out the bad. If any discomfort is experienced, it is generally experienced within the first month. Discomfort is generally in the form of mucus congestion, skin, and digestive or bowel changes. This is normal; it will pass. Simply modify the supplement intake, reducing by half. The foods should remain consistent. Raise the supplements again slowly after the discomfort has disappeared. Make sure you and your children are drinking enough water. Always consult with your family doctor.

Week Three:

Activity 1	Congratulations! You are halfway through your initial program! It's time to assess and re-evaluate. Where have you made progress? In what areas do you want to make more progress? Read through the book to get other ideas about what changes need to be made. Look for support from those you know who have incorporated these ideas in their life. Experiment!!!
Activity 2	Meet with your child or your family to determine how they are adjusting to all these changes. Re-work things accordingly.
Activity 3	It is time to look at dairy products and sugar-containing foods more seriously, if not enough progress has been made. Begin to eliminate all milk products as well as refined sugar products. Foods sweetened with honey, barley malt, or fruit juice may work well. (Consult the Substitution List.)
Activity 4	Continue the good food, the exercise, good water & supplements.
Activity 5	Identify the good fats and bad fats in the diet. Eliminate the bad fats and incorporate the good.
Activity 6	Continue involving the children in menu planning and food preparation.
Activity 7	Have your family make a list of all the harmful chemicals still left in the cupboard, then decide what to do about them.
Activity 8	Take a walk after dinner
Activity 9	Write on your calendar any family member who is ill whether it's a cold, flu, allergies, stomach aches or even one who has an anger outburst. As the weeks go by you may notice less occurrences listed.
Supplements	Continue taking the digestive enzymes supplement. Consider incorporating a probiotic capsule per day, such as acidophilus.
Notice:	Have you noticed a decrease in allergy symptoms -- sinus congestion, clearing the throat, breathing, skin disorders? Have you noticed more consistent bowel movements? Less gas? More balanced moods, balanced energy, and better sleep?

Week Four:

Activity 1	Continue the food, water, and exercise as above.
Activity 2	Utilize whey, rice, or fruit smoothies if there is no time for breakfast or if the children want an after-school snack.
Activity 3	Keep up the good work. You have just changed your children's lives. You have just changed your family's life.
Supplements	Continue the digestive enzymes at one per meal.
	You might find it helpful to add in some cod liver oil by teaspoon or capsule, evening primrose oil by capsule, or flax or hemp oil by teaspoon or capsule. Most kids should have one to two teaspoons per day. Remember that the brain is 60% fat. It will make its membranes out of whatever fats are in the diet.
Results	Time to re-evaluate again. Ask your child or children how they feel and in what areas you and they are looking for more benefit. Instilling body awareness is a "for life" thing. Great work!!!
Notes	Always consult with your family doctor to insure that you are choosing the proper nutritional supplements for your child.

Learn To Ask Important Questions

Instead of Asking:	Ask:
Holding up a can or bottle of soda: Doesn't everyone drink this?	Holding up a can or bottle of soda: Is this beverage regenerating or degenerating? (Does it build or tear down? Does it really feed my child?)
What medicine can I give my child for his or her ear infections, cold, or asthma?	Why is my child getting so many ear infections? Can we prevent them from recurring?
Teachers/School Personnel: Have you thought about putting your child on medication for his or her behavior or learning problem?	Teachers/School Personnel: Have you thought about taking your child to a nutritionist? Have you tried limiting his/her sugar and dairy foods, and cutting out all chemicals, preservatives and additives?
Isn't ADD/ADHD very common now? Aren't prescription drugs the answer?	Why do so many children "have" ADD/ADHD? What are the common denominators? Are there deeper issues? Does the body give us any clues for treatment?
Does this mean we have to live like monks and eat only tofu and bean sprouts?	Are there healthy, good tasting foods to use in place of some of our toxic commercial choices?
Aren't Flintstone vitamins/Centrum vitamins all I need to give my family to insure proper daily nutrient intake?	Can we really get all we need from one multi-vitamin? How can I customize our nutrition program for what my child needs?

Simple Substitutions

7-up	Zevia Lemon Lime Soda
Captain Crunch	Gorilla Munch (gluten free)
Cheerios	Oatios or Kamutios (New Morning)
Cheetos	Cheese Puffs (Barbara's)
Coke, Pepsi, Or Diet	Dr. Tima's Honey Cola, Blue Sky Cola, 365 cola, Natural Brew Draft Cola
Commercial Pizza	Make your own: Foccacia crust kids love to choose toppings, Brown Rice Crust Pizza (Nature's Hilights) Spelt Crust Pizza (Grainassance)
Commercial Potato Chips	Boulder Chips, Barbara's Potato Chips
Corn Flakes	Kamut, Quinoa, Amaranth Flakes (New Morning)
Egg beaters	Eggs or Egg Replacer
Eggo frozen waffles	Van's organic frozen waffles (regular, blueberry, or wheat-free) Trader Joe's
Flavored Oatmeal Pkts.	Real oatmeal with Sucanat, honey, jam
Gatorade	Recharge or Emergen C, Clif Kid Splashers
Ginger Ale	Reed's Ginger Brew, 365 Ginger Ale
Hershey's chocolate bar	Baker's German Sweet Chocolate Bar, many brands of organic chocolate
Hot chocolate	Ah, Alaska (99% caffeine-free)
Imitation vanilla (vanillin)	Pure vanilla extract
Jell-o	Knox unflavored gelatin + org. fruit juice
Kool-Aid	1 cup organic fruit juice, 2 cups water
M&M's	Sunspire Sundrops (plain & peanut)
Macaroni and Cheese	Annie's or De Boles Macaroni and Cheese (boxed)
Milk	Organic milk (Horizon) or Rice Dream, hemp milk, almond milk, or mix all
Miracle Whip or Mayonnaises	Nayonaise (egg-free), Vegenaise (with grape seed oil, no egg), many other varieties of spreads (Spectrum Naturals, Hain)
Quaker Choc, Chip Granola Bars	Healthy Valley Chocolate Chip Granola Bars
Rice Crispies	Brown Rice Crispies
Spaghettio's	Grandma Millina's Pasta Rings (w/Veggie Franks)
Sugar, Nutrasweet	Sucanat or Stevia drops or powder
Toothpastes with dye & artificial flavoring	Desert Essence, Nutrabiotic, others

Food Diary

Use this chart to track your child's food intake.

Name ______________________________ Date: __________

	Day 1	Day 2	Day 3	Day 4	Day 5	Day 6	Day 7
Breakfast							
Symptoms							
Lunch							
Symptoms							
Dinner							
Symptoms							
Snacks- note time							
Symptoms							

Weighing Quality and Price of Natural Foods & Supplements

A common question that many people ask is, how much does it cost to make all these changes in the diet and add supplements to the family regime as well? Can we afford this?

Here is my answer. When I walk through health food stores, I see people who are from many different income levels. Some are affluent and some are not. How do they do it? They have **prioritized health in their lives**. They have decided to spend more money on their food and supplements and less on other things like Starbuck's coffee and a scone, or cigarettes or gummy bears. Somehow, when you have a goal that you're focusing on, everything works out.

- Construct a health program according to your budget. Maybe you can start with everything at once, or maybe you'll need to take incremental steps. In other words, build the program slowly, until you see what you can handle financially.
- When you begin to eat simple, fresh foods, you buy fewer packaged foods. Packaged foods are expensive. Making this switch is more time-consuming for the cook, but well worth the payoff on the other end.
- Buy in bulk from the health food store. The bulk bins in most stores offer "loose" grains, cereals, mixes, nuts and seeds. The price is reduced because the foods are not packaged. Many health food cereal equivalents to mainstream cereals can be found in this bulk section: healthier "cheerios", flakes, puffs and granolas.
- Purchase your favorite items by the case and get a discount. Rice milk, soups and spring water can be stored for weeks. (You can place a special order.)
- Reduce consumption of most beverages, except pure water. When you eliminate soda and juice drinking, some of your expenses are cut. Many kids do just fine on water primarily, with an occasional juice or health food soda as a treat. Some herb teas, sweetened at home with stevia can be served iced or hot and taste great. Moms remark about how it has saved them on a hot summer day. And the great thing is that after drinking it, the child has no blood sugar reaction because stevia does not cause the insulin surge that other sweeteners do.
- If you have very little money, not enough to start a supplement program, then first work with eliminating all the artificial substances from your family's diet: preservatives, additives, artificial sweeteners and food colorings. This is a start.

- If you only have enough money to start a minimal supplement program, then begin with one supplement of choice and use it for one to three months. Then switch to another and continue to rotate. Baby steps are better than none at all.
- Get together with a friend or group of people to create your own "co-op". You can purchase items by the case at a discount. Divide it up and split the cost.
- **People also ask: can I buy the supplements at low cost pharmacies, grocery stores or special warehouse stores?** Most supplements from the health food stores, network marketing companies and your health practitioners are of better quality than those you buy at low cost pharmacies or grocery stores. The raw materials are most often scrutinized for purity and quality by these companies. They have a vested interest in the beneficial and therapeutic outcome of the products they offer, as they communicate generally on a one-to-one basis with the customer and depend on their repeat business. More importantly, they have studied the field and have more expert opinions on health than most sales people in grocery stores.

In order for change to happen, you have to make a change.
That may necessitate starting with a change in mental attitude and a willingness to embrace the concept that we can and should take control of our own health.
It is our birthright: it is free.

~ ~ ~

Chapter Fifteen

OUR SCHOOLS & COMMUNITY: An Action Plan

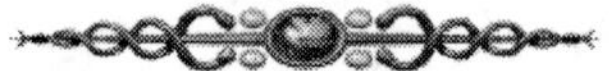

How Parents Can Help

The greatest impact on children's health usually starts at home, with the parents. Here are suggestions for keeping your family in tip-top shape:

Getting Acquainted with Nutritional Information

- Educate yourselves about the many natural approaches for helping with learning and behavior problems with children.
    - Go to educational seminars about nutrition as well as behavior modification and other alternatives.
    - Read, listen to CD's, and watch informative videos and DVD's.
    - Network. Talk with other parents who have found success with natural methods.
    - Speak with a nutritionist, a chiropractor, a psychologist, a neurofeedback specialist who has had success with children.
- In family meetings and conversations, educate your children about good nutritional practices and chemical-free, healthy foods.
- Create activities around label-reading. Teach your kids to read labels in the store, when shopping. Emphasize that chemicals are harmful.

Creating Activities: Food and Your Kitchen

- Cook at home as much as possible. You have control over the quality of ingredients and energetics of your food.
- Eat at least one meal daily together.
- Teach portion control to your kids. If you use small plates, portions will be smaller.

Tips to help you and your child with portion sizes.

1. A 1/2 cup serving of fruit, vegetables, or potatoes looks like half a tennis ball sitting on your plate.
2. 3 ounces of meat, fish, or chicken is about the size of a deck of playing cards or the palm of your hand.
3. A 1 ounce serving of cheese is about the size of your thumb.

4. A 1 cup serving of milk, yogurt, or fresh greens is about the size of your fist.
5. 1 teaspoon of oil is about the size of your thumb tip

- Wait 10-15 minutes before going back for seconds.
- Encourage your children to cook or help prepare some of their own food. Depending on the age, they can create or just stir.
- Give the child his or her own cabinet and utensils.
- Keep snack foods in ziploc bags so they are not as accessible.
- Include your child in menu planning.
- Be creative with restricted diets. There is a whole world of foods out there. For variety, think multi-cultural foods; collect recipes.
- Be creative with names for food. Call a milkshake "Nuclear Waste Sludge".
- Communicate with your child about whether he or she is enjoying the food? Offer choices. Bargaining is O.K.

Trying Nutritional Supplements

- Emphasize the importance of taking supplements. By nature, kids ask, "why?" List the positive benefits, such as better energy, clearer skin, increased strength and speed in sports.
- Do experiments: open a digestive enzyme capsule into a cup of pudding. Watch it liquefy, demonstrating how enzymes digest food.
- Some parents say the best time to emphasize the importance of taking supplements is when the child is sick. Everyone wants to feel good, and children who are nutritionally replete have fewer colds and flues.
- Don't make faces or hold your nose while putting his/her capsules into juice or food. Respect the new diet/program.
- If a child responds that having to take supplements and eat certain foods is unfair, reinforce that life sometimes is unfair, but there is always an "up-side". The glass is half-full most of the time and half-empty the others.
- Give them a choice: "Do you want your acidophilus at breakfast or your digestive enzymes?"
- Feed vitamins or algae plant food to your houseplants or garden. Remark how it helps them grow faster and stronger.
- Feed your pets supplements. Ask your children to participate in the feeding.

Getting Involved in Health Activities

- Encourage kids with ADD/ADHD to get involved in non-competitive sports.
- Take a family walk after dinner each night.

- Challenge your kids to a jumping jack contest during T.V. commercials.
- Encourage creativity in music and art as viable ways of self-expression. Many ADHD kids are very artistic. Playing Mozart and Bach can help create an environment conducive to learning as well as peace. (See Resources List.)
- Communicate with the teachers about the information and research you have discovered. What we eat does effect our emotions, behavior and attitudes. Show them the research in this book.
- If a child gets sugar or chemical-laden foods as snacks/prizes from their teacher, ask them to bring the candy/food home and for every piece they bring home, you buy them a natural food candy.
- Ask the teachers to participate in educating about natural health and nutrition.
- Invite a teacher for a protein drink like the one's you and your kids drink – a green drink or a whey protein shake in the morning or at a coffee break. Put information in the teachers' lounge about nutrition and the brain.
- Find another parent with a child who's a friend of your child --- and ask that they become involved in this nutritional "project" with you.
- Appreciate the new world of food that's opening up and the potential a new diet and/or supplement protocol has for changing your lives.

BE AN EXAMPLE. Only ask a child to do something you would be willing to do. Be patient. Trust the process.

How Teachers Can Help

Teachers, today, have a long "to do" list. I don't know how they get everything done. It's commendable. The suggestions below may add to their "to do" list, but in the long run, the improvement in the students' behavior and school performance will more than compensate for their time and efforts.

Assist in Your Students' Health

- Encourage naturally-sweetened snacks, without sugar or artificial sweeteners.
- Encourage chemical-free snacks, without colorings, preservatives, and additives.
    - trail mix, nuts, seeds (Have the kids mix their favorite combo.)
    - rice cakes with fruit spread and almond butter
    - apples, bananas, grapes, pears, oranges and tangerines
    - unsweetened fruit juices
    - tomato or carrot juice

- vegetable sticks

- Offer non-food rewards for special achievements. Give points that accumulate toward a pick of a "prize box", containing key chains, pencils, small toys.
- Reward your students with special activities that they like, rather than food.
- Take your nutritional supplements in front of the kids, (according to school policies). Drink green drinks.
- Put plants in your classroom to catch the air-born phenols and clean the air. The best plants for air-cleaning are spider plants, Boston fern, English ivy and palms.
- Avoid wearing commercial perfumes, as many ADHD children, asthmatics and children with allergies are sensitive to the chemicals in the perfume.

Be Part of a Valuable Support System

- Interact with parents about learning and behavior progress of their children.
- Observe physical reactions: red ears, red cheeks, and rashes ---- reactions to foods. Report these to the parents, as they are clues to sensitivities that can result in cognitive or behavioral changes.
- Educate yourself about the many natural approaches that people have had great success with, such as nutrition, chiropractic, and neurofeedback. Talk with doctors and health practitioners who are having success with drug-free programs.
- Suggest to the parent: "There is fascinating new research on the effects of chemicals, preservatives, and colorings in food and how they relate to health and behavior." Show them the studies in this book.

Create Projects

- Integrate nutritional information into core subjects, such as science, history and language arts. Educate your classes about the importance of nutrient-rich foods.
- Carry on sprouting projects or grow herbs in the classroom.
- Participate in school or community garden projects.
- Give away tomato seedlings in the spring. The students' task is to grow them at home during the summer. Have a contest for biggest, reddest and funniest, when kids come back in the fall. Kids write of their tomato experience.
- Take a field trip to your local health food store. (www.fieldtripfactory.com.)
- Spread the word to other teachers, counselors, and administrators. Speak at special parent education classes.

How School Officials & Personnel Can Be Supportive

Commitment at the highest level of school leadership is essential for implementing a strong health program. Schools play an important role in children's lives and can do more than any other institution to promote lifetime health. Children spend much of their time in the school setting and are impacted by the environment, for better or worse.

The Surgeon General released a "call to action" encouraging schools to join a nationwide effort to prevent overweight and obesity. Schools can take the following action steps to ensure children's health and academic success:

- Provide a quality nutrition and physical education program that helps students develop the knowledge and behaviors to enjoy healthy eating habits and a physically active lifestyle.
- Encourage the PTA committees to create awareness about nutrition as it relates to learning and behavior. Bring in qualified speakers who specialize in these areas.
- Provide training on healthy cooking techniques for cafeteria staff. (Videos, CD-ROM's, or a health food culinary expert)
- Encourage the health personnel to be knowledgeable about nutritional, as well as environmental health.
- Expand the nutrition and health sections in the school libraries.

Take Action with Food and the Environment

- Explore creative ways to improve the quality of food selections:
- Develop within the curriculum-- high school, alternative school, middle school -- a greenhouse management program. Grow various sprouts of vegetables, nuts, beans, lentils, grains and seeds to provide live, organic, diverse, healthy food choices that are added to cafeteria salad bars daily.
- Develop a seed/life appreciation/sprout curriculum early that allows children to grow organic sprouts for their daily snacking. Include nuts, seeds, beans, lentils and grains.
- Eliminate candy and "junk food" from vending machines. Replace with fruit and trail mixes.
- Eliminate soda pop from vending machines. Replace with bars dispensing fresh juice, or organic fruit or vegetable juices without sucrose. Water is good option.
- Eliminate BHA, BHT, preservatives and food coloring from school foods. (Check *Chapter 4* for scientific references.)

- Encourage your community to provide well-maintained and close-to-home sidewalks, bike paths, trails and recreation facilities.
- Investigate the use of non-toxic lawn and outdoor products.
- Help teachers make their classrooms environmentally safe, cleaned with products that are better tolerated by sensitive individuals, and carpet-free. Invest in full-spectrum lighting, as conventional lights can cause focus and behavior problems.
- Encourage students and teachers to appreciate food as it relates to their health.
- Sign your school up for the "President's Challenge" for fun physical activities. There are many companies and organizations that support the President's Challenge campaign by donating sports equipment, grants or educational materials if you participate. ***Take the Challenge!*** www.presidentschallenge.org

What Communities Can Do

Make Healthy Choices Easy

- Come together to encourage families to eat home more and buy natural foods from the grocery stores, natural food stores and farmers' markets.
- Create opportunities for a variety of enjoyable, confidence-instilling physical activities for children and teens. Involve friends, peers and parents.
- Provide daily K - 12 physical education classes. Hire physical education specialists to teach them. They will be good role models as well.
- Provide access to school buildings and community facilities that enable safe participation in physical activity.
- Encourage health care providers to talk routinely to adolescents and teens about how to eat smart and incorporate physical activity into their lives.

Help People Adopt Healthy Lifestyles

- Design communities that are "walk-able".
- Implement safe routes to school programs, plant trees and create public gardens. Form partnerships among local governments, business leaders and policymakers to work together to deliberately plan for smart community growth to promote health.

Implement Affordable and Healthful Food Options

- Community leaders and policymakers can create business incentives to increase access to healthy foods in underserved communities. Start farmers' markets and develop delivery systems to provide low-cost fresh fruits and vegetables to families at after-school care programs and worksites. Some farmers' markets offer cooking and nutrition lessons to help consumers choose and prepare healthy foods.

Emphasize the Importance of Health in the Workplace

- Employers can provide healthy food choices in cafeterias and vending machines.
- Employers can offer opportunities for physical activity. One company has a great idea – they pop a yoga and Pilate's tape in at 5 pm and interested employees do yoga together before they go home.
- Bring in local health practitioners - like chiropractors to educate employees about how proper physical alignment can help de-stress and eliminate pain.
- Bring in nutritionists and naturopaths to help educate employees about how to prevent colds, flues, and allergies. This will increase work attendance and build morale. Many of the employees are parents and they'll teach their children.
- Offer HSA's or Health Savings Accounts that cover alternative health care solutions that insurance companies do not.

Encourage Physical Activity Time in Schools and Day Care Centers

- Communities can encourage local school districts to require physical education in elementary schools.
- Encourage local YMCAs to implement physical activity in after-school child care programs.
- Monitor progress of the students and the success of programs put into place by Body Mass Index Monitoring. A simple chart is used to compare a child's weight by height against the "norm" on the chart. When done yearly, this can help decrease the prevalence of childhood obesity by increasing awareness.

What Legislators Can Do

- Take action to make wholesome, natural food more accessible in schools.
- Lawmakers can ensure that health consequences are weighed in legislative and regulatory decisions that impact community structure.
- Raise standards for health and physical education in the classroom.
- Enact policies that encourage the location of new schools in areas where students can safely walk or bike. Support improving the condition of aging school buildings.

- Be a champion for health in your community. Hometown leaders and lawmakers can help change lives with the decisions they make.

Other resources:
www.aahperd.org/naspe
www.actionforhealthykids.org
www.cdc.gov/nccdphp/dnpa/kidswalk
www.kidseatwell.org
www.presidentshchallenge.org
www.school-lunch.org
www.walktoschool.org

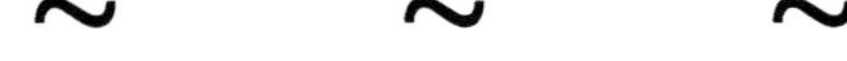

IMPORTANT RESOURCES LIST

Experts

Peter Breggin, M.D.: Dr. Breggin has been called "the conscience of psychiatry" for his efforts to reform the mental health field, including his promotion of caring psychotherapeutic approaches and his opposition to the escalating overuse of psychiatric medications, the oppressive diagnosing and drugging of children, electroshock, lobotomy, involuntary treatment, and false biological theories.
www.breggin.com

John Taylor, PhD: Dr. Taylor is the founder and president of ADD-Plus. He is widely regarded as an innovator and pioneering authority in the field of Attention Deficit Disorders. He is the author of thirteen books, including 'Helping Your ADD Child', over 200 articles in journals and professional newsletters, and numerous educational resource materials used internationally.
www.ADD-Plus.com 800-847-1233

Gluten and Casein-Free Food

www.arrowheadmills.com
www.celiac.com
www.gfcfdiet.com
www.gfmall.com
www.glutenfreeinfo.com
www.glutenfreemall.com
www.glutenfreeoats.com
www.glutino.com
www.specialfoods.com
www.sylvanborderfarm.com
www.vancesfoods.com
www.wholefoodsmarket.com

Authentic Foods: Bean flour, bean flour mixes and other baking supplies
www.authenticfoods.com

Bob's Red Mill Natural Foods, Inc: Wheat and gluten free flours
www.bobsredmill.com

Cause You're Special Company: Mixes and baking supplies
www.causeyourespecial.com

Dietary Specialties, Inc: Flours, mixes, pasta, crackers, cookies & condiments
www.dietspec.com

Ener-G-Foods, Inc: Flours, baking supplies, baked goods
www.ener-g.com

Gillian's Foods: Rolls and other products
www.gilliansfoods.com

Glutano Ltd: Breads, cakes, cereals, cookies
www.glutenfree-foods.co.uk

Gluten-Free Pantry: Mixes, pasta, baking supplies
www.glutenfree.com

Jules Gluten-Free: All purpose gluten-free flour and newsletter
www.julesglutenfree.com

Kingsmill Foods, Inc: Breads, cookies
www.kingsmillfoods.com

Kinnikinnick Foods, Inc: Ice cream cones, crispy rice, cereal, baked goods
www.kinnikinnick.com

Miss Roben's, Inc: Gluten-free mixes, pasta, baking supplies, good newsletter
www.allergygrocer.com

Roma Food Products: Gluten-free, egg-free cookies, pastas, flours, mixes
www.orgran.com

Shiloh Farms: Gluten-free cereals, flours and snacks
http://www.shilohfarms.com

Laboratories for Testing

Diagnos-Techs: Complete intestinal pathogen analysis and digestive markers with stool samples. Food antibodies and hormonal testing through the saliva.
www.diagnostechs.com

Doctor's Data: Routine Chemistry, Toxicology, Bacteriology, Mycology, Parasitology, and General Immunology.
www.DoctorsData.com

Entero Lab: Testing for specific food sensitivities, the most comprehensive gluten testing, genetic gluten testing.
www.enterolab.com

Genova Diagnostics: (formerly Great Smokey Labs, Inc) Clinical chemistry, Bacteriology, Mycology, Parasitology, Virology, Microbiology, General Immunology, Hematology, Toxicology, as well as Molecular Genetics.
www.genovadiagnostics.com

Immunosciences Lab: Comprehensive, specific immunological testing.
www.immunoscience.com

MetaMetrix Lab: Recognized internationally as a leader in the development of nutritional, metabolic and toxicant testing. Organic acid, amino acid and fatty acid analyses, detoxification markers, nutrient markers, gut pathogens.
www.metametrix.com

Neurosciences: Neurological, Endocrinological & Immunological Assessments
www.neurorelief.com

Sabre Sciences: Leader on the cutting edge in the field of Endocrinology. Dedicated to comprehensive hormonal and neuroendocrine health. Male, female and child hormone and neurotransmitter testing. Customized Cream Formulations.
www.sabresciences.com

Miscellaneous

www.aahperd.org/naspe - National Assoc. for Sport and Physical Education
www.actionforhealthykids.org
www.ajcn.org/cgi/content/full/76/1/5/T1 (glycemic index & glycemic load charts)
www.campmor.com (safer drinking water containers)
www.cdc.gov/nccdphp/dnpa/kidswalk
www.fieldtripfactory.com
www.iabdm and www.iaomt.org (holistic or biological dentistry)
www.kidseatwell.org
www.ourchildrenshealth.com/guidelines (health questionnaire)
www.presidentschallenge.org
www.school-lunch.org
www.walktoschool.org

Nutritional Supplements

www.detoxamin.com (chelation supplements)

www.scicn.com Other Nutritional Supplements: Southern California Institute of Clinical Nutrition, 800-608-5602

www.simplexityhealth.com Simplexity Health (Super Blue Green Algae): 800-800-1300

Organizations

www.ajcn.org (American Journal of Clinical Nutrition)
www.bulimia.com
www.celiac.com
www.celiac.org
www.celiaccentral.org
www.chadd.org
www.csaceliacs.org
www.nvic.org (National Vaccine Information Center)
www.safeminds.org

The Feingold Association: believes that patients have a right to be given complete, accurate information on all of the options available in the treatment of ADHD as well as other conditions. Sometimes, the best results come from a combination of treatments. This might include using the Feingold Diet plus allergy treatments, or plus nutritional supplements, or plus a gluten-free/casein-free diet, or even Feingold + ADHD medicine. It's useful to start with the Feingold Diet since it is fairly easy to use, not expensive, and because removing certain synthetic additives is a good idea for anyone.
www.feingold.org 800-321-3287

Recommended Reading/Listening

Essential Gluten-Free Dining Guide, published by Triumph Din

Fact'R and ADD+ Catalogue of Books and Tapes for parents and Professionals - Dr. John Taylor, call: 800-847-1233.

Kids with Celiac Disease: A Family Guide to Raising Happy, Healthy, Gluten-Free Children, by Danna Korn, one of the foremost experts on gluten-free living
Listening with the Whole Body, by Sheila M Frick

Excellent resource, especially for the autistic spectrum. Lays the foundation for the mechanics of eating.

Living Gluten-Free for Dummies, by Danna Korn
Practical, friendly guide to successfully managing a gluten-free diet.

Sound Bodies through Sound Therapy, by Dorinne S. Davis
Good foundation book about how the auditory system works and a description of the different therapies including Bioacoustics.

The Great Defender: Your Immune System – investigative reporter, Jon Rappoport interviews Dr. Laura Thompson. CD www.scicn.com

The Out-of-Sync Child: Recognizing and Coping with Sensory Processing Disorder, Revised Edition, by Carol Stock Kranowitz
Lots of charts and checklists

Vaccination Resources List

The following websites contain vaccine exemption forms per state, vaccine ingredients, vaccine studies that we don't hear about:

www.lewrockwell.com/miller/miller15.html (user-friendly vaccine schedule)
www.newmediaexplorer.org/sepp (global vaccine info updates)
www.nmaseminars.com (Dr. Sherri Tenpenny + "just say no" blog)
www.nvic.org/state-site/state-exemptions.htm (state laws and exemptions, ingredient list, myths and facts)
www.ourchildrenshealth.com (chart of excipients & ingredients)
www.thenhf.com/vaccinations.html
www.vaclib.org (what every parent should know)

Conventional vaccine info websites:
www.cdc.gov/vaccines (Centers for Disease Control)
www.cispimmunize.org (American Academy of Pediatrics)
www.immunizationinfo.org/vaccineInfo/index.cfm#state (National Network for Immunization Information)

Books:
"A Shot in the Dark", co-authored by Harris Coulter and National Vaccine Information Center President and Co-founder, Barbara Loe Fisher, who helped launch the vaccine safety and informed consent movement.

"FOWL! Bird Flu: It's Not What You Think", by Dr. Sherri J. Tenpenny examines mandatory vaccination and discusses the relationship between pharmaceutical and chemical companies and agribusiness.

"Saying 'No' To Vaccines:" A Resource Guide for All Ages, Dr. Sherri J. Tenpenny

"Vaccinations: A Thoughtful Parents' Guide", discusses your vaccine choices, benefits, risk and alternatives.

"Vaccine Guide: Risks and Benefits for Children and Adults" (Paperback), by Randall Neustaedter

*"Vaccines: The Risks, the Benefits, the Choices, a Resource Guide for Parents" (*Paperback), by Dr. Sherri J. Tenpenny

"What Every Parent Should Know About Childhood Immunizations", by Jamie Murphy, reviews information on childhood vaccines and examines the effect of vaccines on the immune system.

"What Your Doctor May Not Tell You About Children's Vaccinations", by Dr. Stephanie Cave, is a down-to-earth guide to help you make vaccination choices.

Index

N

O

P

R

S

T

V

W

X

Z